21-DAY
Tummy

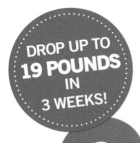

DROP UP TO
19 POUNDS
IN
3 WEEKS!

**Target Dangerous Fat
and Digestive Discomfort
In One Delicious Plan**

21-DAY
Tummy

THE REVOLUTIONARY DIET
THAT SOOTHES AND SHRINKS
ANY BELLY FAST

BY **LIZ VACCARIELLO**

Author of the *New York Times* Bestseller *The Digest Diet*

WITH **KATE SCARLATA, RD**

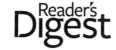

Reader's
Digest

The Reader's Digest Association, Inc.
New York, NY/Montreal

A READER'S DIGEST BOOK
Copyright © 2013 The Reader's Digest Association, Inc.
All rights reserved. Unauthorized reproduction, in any manner, is prohibited.
Reader's Digest is a registered trademark of The Reader's Digest Association, Inc.

Food photographs by Andrew Purcell
Test team photographs by Steve Vaccariello
Exercise illustrations by Jason Lee

Clothing for test team provided by Old Navy, Target, and Kohl's.

LIBRARY OF CONGRESS CATALOGING-IN-PUBLICATION DATA
Vaccariello, Liz, author.
   21-day tummy : the revolutionary food plan that shrinks and soothes any belly fast / Liz
Vaccariello, author of the New York Times bestsellers Flat belly diet! and The Digest diet, with
Kate Scarlata, RD.
        pages cm
   Includes bibliographical references and index.
   ISBN 978-1-62145-111-2 (alk. paper) -- ISBN 978-1-62145-113-6 (epub)
   1. Reducing diets--Recipes. 2. Diet therapy. 3. Menus. I. Scarlata, Kate, author. II. Title. III.
Title: Twenty-one-day tummy.
   RM222.2.V246 2013
   641.5'635--dc23
                                        2013021145

ISBN 978-1-62145-111-2

We are committed to both the quality of our products and the service we provide to our
customers. We value your comments, so please feel free to contact us.

        The Reader's Digest Association, Inc.
        Adult Trade Publishing
        44 South Broadway
        White Plains, NY 10601

For more Reader's Digest products and information, visit our website:
        www.rd.com (in the United States)
        www.readersdigest.ca (in Canada)

Printed in the United States of America

1 3 5 7 9 10 8 6 4 2

NOTE TO OUR READERS

The information in this book should not be substituted for, or used to alter, medical therapy
without your doctor's advice. For a specific health problem, consult your physician for guidance.

Contents

Acknowledgements

To serve as the editor-in-chief and chief content officer of Reader's Digest is a dream come true. I thank CEO Bob Guth for the opportunity and the resources to further the mission of this beloved brand, which is to simplify and enrich our readers' lives. My gratitude also to Marilynn Jacobs and Harold Clarke, who believed in the potential of this book from the very beginning.

I have been blessed to work with some of the most creative and hardest-working people in the business, including executive editor and friend Courtenay Smith and dynamo design director Dean Abatemarco, whose guidance has been instrumental in elevating the quality of everything we publish. Thanks also to Lauren Gelman, Perri O. Blumberg, Lauren Stine, Elizabeth Kelly, and Adrienne Farr for their work supporting the creation of this book.

I have to give a special shout-out to Rebecca Simpson Steele, the brilliant photo editor who dreamed up a theme that made both our food and our testers shine. Thanks to her team, Emilie Harjes and Alexa Speyer. And of course, to our photographers—my better half, Steve Vaccariello, who always makes me feel like a rock star and did the same for all our panelists; and Andrew Purcell, who made our recipes look every bit as appetizing as they taste. And to the stylists: Elysha Lenkin; Nikki Wang; Margie Bresciani and Amy Klewitz of Pro-Style-Crew; and Carrie Purcell and Sarah Cave of Big Leo.

My gratitude also to Marti Golon and Jason Lee, for the easy-to-follow exercise illustrations. And to Diane Dragan and the video team, who captured the success of our test panel so well: Nick Montalvo, Dino Castelli, Herman Tang, Peter Tooke, and Tani Alvarez.

To the amazing Reader's Digest book team, which creates fresh, dynamic, life-enriching books under incredible deadlines: senior editor Andrea Au Levitt, design director George McKeon, and managing editor Lorraine Burton. Special thanks also to Jen Tokarski, Susan Hindman, Laura C. Wood, and Nan Badgett. Without them, this book would not have been made.

Fist bumps to my fellow test panelists: Jonathan Bigham, Tonya Carkeet, Adrienne Farr, Phyllis Gebhardt, Jaimie Hoffman, Rob

McMahon, Sabrina Ng, Dorothy Nuzzo, Kate Rattner, Gregg Roth, and Lauren Weiss. And thanks to Mindy Hermann, RD, for weighing and measuring everyone with an encouraging smile.

And of course, this book would not be complete without the efforts of Michele Stanten, who created the exercise program, and Kate Slate and Sandy Gluck, who developed the delicious recipes. I owe a debt of gratitude to registered dietitian and plan creator Kate Scarlata, RD, LDN, who went above and beyond the call of duty to answer testers' questions (including mine!), review countless versions of the manuscript, and develop a menu that is delicious and works miracles! Thank you, thank you, thank you!

Finally, I'd like to thank my family for joining me in this adventure. Lori, for helping cook and measure, then measure and cook again. And Steve, Olivia, and Sophia for everything, always.

Introduction

In my decades as a health journalist, I've watched the evidence pile up: Weight is intimately connected to health. That's why, when I run across research that can help people get to their healthiest weight, I want to get it in the hands of as many people as possible. When I first saw the Spanish study that indicated you could target dangerous belly fat by eating more monounsaturated fatty acids (MUFAs), I wrote *Flat Belly Diet!* When I learned that scientists had targeted even more foods and nutrients that could help you release fat, I brought you *The Digest Diet.* But when I stumbled upon research linking two of my own personal challenges, weight gain and digestive slowdown, I knew I had a fresh solution to yet another unique problem.

I've gotta say, I'm a little nervous writing about my . . . issues. As the editor-in-chief of *Reader's Digest,* I've grown used to sharing details of my private life in my monthly editor's notes. But nothing I write there is as personal as what I'll be sharing here.

Constipation.

Halfway through my 40s, I noticed some subtle changes in the way my body worked. At the same time I was becoming less and less regular, I also suffered from almost constant bloating, and endured severe cramping after I ate. On top of that, I'd gained almost 10 pounds! Technically, I was in a healthy weight range, but I felt like I carried a heavy belly balloon around. My clothes didn't fit. The discomfort was constant and distracting.

As I watched the scale creep up a pound or two every few months despite my healthy diet and faithfully active lifestyle, it was time to consider the factors at work. First, there is our good friend Father Time. As we get older, we naturally lose muscle mass, our metabolism slows, and maintaining weight becomes tougher. At 45, thanks to my devotion to weight training, that wasn't a major factor for me. I had a different setback to contend with: forced inactivity. A recent bunion surgery left me immobile for more than a month: bedridden for 2 weeks, then confined to sitting for another 4. This was tough, since I'm an avid mover and am used to walking an hour a day. Being immobilized not only made me feel stuck but also put the pounds on.

Remember, I'm not fat. I believe the pursuit of "skinny" is vapid and unhealthy. What I do want, though, is to be at a weight where I feel my best. A heavier, distended midsection made that impossible.

The more I started talking about my digestive challenges, the more people confided their own private struggles. From burps and groans to discomfort and moans, millions of Americans have tummy issues. One of the most common? Extra weight. With that weight frequently comes indigestion, painful stomach cramps, or an uncomfortable bloated feeling. These problems are annoying but often don't seem serious enough to mention to a doctor. Maybe you pop some antacids and call it a day. Or, if you suspect that you have gluten or lactose intolerance, you may (needlessly) cut whole food groups out of your diet. It was a real eureka moment for me when I finally made a discovery that would change my body and my life: The foods that lead

> From burps and groans to discomfort and moans, millions of Americans have stomach issues.

to gastrointestinal (GI) problems are often the same ones that pack on the pounds. Of course, the flip side is also true: The same diet that leads to a trim tummy also solves several common GI problems, including heartburn and acid reflux, gas and bloating, constipation, diarrhea, and irritable bowel syndrome (IBS). That's right. It's possible to lose weight and improve digestion at the same time. This book will show you how.

At Reader's Digest, we have a long history (90-plus years!) of finding the best and most cutting-edge medical science, and curating and condensing it so that it's most useful. That's exactly what we've done with *21-Day Tummy*. My team and I sought out all the latest research on both weight loss and digestive issues (there proved to be a lot of it!). While dietitians, doctors, and GI sufferers have long suspected a connection between what's going on in your gut and the rest of your body, science is only now beginning to catch up. This is currently a hot topic for research and we uncovered reams of pioneering studies, many of which upended my notions of what's good for weight loss and health.

For the all-important layer of dietary expertise, I sought out Kate Scarlata, a registered dietitian who specializes in treating patients with digestive disorders. Kate has 25 years of experience in the nutrition and wellness field, including seven years at Harvard-affiliated Brigham and Women's Hospital. As someone who has experienced digestive issues herself,

Kate has made it her business to stay on top of the research about what really troubles your tummy. But she also knows we don't live in a laboratory; for any eating plan to work, it needs to be one you can follow in the real world. Combining the revolutionary science with her patients' successes, she created a plan that first eliminates all your digestive issues, while simultaneously trimming your belly. Then, as you lose weight, she helps you identify your own trigger foods so your tummy stays slim and calm for life. Kate has been my savior. And now she can be yours, too!

The 21-Day Tummy diet works. How do I know?

Because I did it myself and I lost 10 pounds in 3 weeks. More important: I feel 100 percent healthy. My symptoms disappeared almost immediately and I haven't seen them since! Now that I know what my particular problem foods are, I can avoid them. That way, I remain lean, healthy, and happy: My digestion problems are a thing of the past, and so is that extra pooch.

To round out the experience, I recruited 11 colleagues, friends, and readers to try the diet with me. The grand tally of our weight loss in 3 weeks: 90 pounds! Our testers shed 29 inches collectively from their waists (that's a lot of belly fat!), and every one of them reported improved digestion.

My colleague Rob McMahon was our biggest weight-loss success story, shedding a whopping 19 pounds in just 21 days—a feat made all the more impressive when you consider that he was traveling (both for business and on vacation) and having to eat out for many of those days. Also, Rob was able to completely stop taking acid reflux medication, something he had become dependent on to get through the day without pain. You'll read more about Rob's story—and all our other testers' successes—throughout the book.

I'm amazed at how great eating this way makes me feel. I'm sleeping like a baby, I'm bounding with energy, my skin has taken on a glow, and I swear my hair is growing faster (is that possible?). But the best part? My digestion is regular, and I don't feel crampy and bloated anymore. I've always eaten healthfully, but this specific combination of high-magnesium, low-sugar, high-fiber, and carb-light foods works for my system in a way I've never felt before. God willing, I've found my solution.

> I recruited 11 people to try the diet with me. The grand tally of our weight loss in 3 weeks: 90 pounds!

The way to soothe and shrink your stomach is to do two things—**balance gut flora** (the bacteria in our GI tract) and **reduce inflammation.** To do this, the 21-Day Tummy plan has you follow four food rules. You will eat:

1. More magnesium-rich foods

2. More anti-inflammatory fats

3. Fewer carb-dense foods

4. Fewer FODMAPs (These are carbs, mostly sugars, that ferment rapidly. More about them later.)

It's easier to think of these foods in two categories: Belly Buddies, which help soothe the digestive system, calm inflammation, and shrink fat cells; and Belly Bullies, which can cause indigestion, inflammation, and bloating. You'll avoid the Belly Bullies (like milk, high fructose sugars, and wheat) and embrace the Belly Buddies (including everyday favorites such as peanut butter, bananas, and Greek yogurt). The plan is not only easy to follow but delicious!

If you've read any of my previous books, you know how much I love food. So in order for me to stand behind any diet plan, it needs to feature scrumptious, real foods that are easy for a busy working mom like me to cook. You'll find more than 50 yummy 21-Day Tummy recipes in the book—including my faves Tomato-Ginger Flank Steak, Curry-Rubbed Chicken with Fresh Pineapple Chutney, and Hearty Roasted Vegetable Soup—in addition to the many quick-fix meals in the 21-day meal plan.

And since I know from personal experience that exercise is also key to a lean look, I included an equipment-free workout that's specially designed to complement the 21-Day Tummy diet. Not only does it sculpt and strengthen your core muscles in as little as 15 minutes a day, it incorporates ab fat–torching interval walks to trim your tummy and stress-busting yoga poses to calm it.

The 21-Day Tummy diet is a weight loss program that can help anyone shed belly fat in just 3 weeks. But what makes it unique, and distinct from anything else out there, is its ability to treat, and sometimes even cure, the five most common digestive disorders: heartburn and acid reflux, gas and bloating, constipation, diarrhea, and IBS. If you suffer from other GI issues, like ulcerative colitis, Crohn's disease, or other types of inflammatory bowel disease (IBD), you may also find relief on *21-Day Tummy*. Please consult your doctor first, since those conditions require individualized treatment plans managed by a physician, nurse practitioner, and/or registered dietitian. Similarly, this diet may help prevent gallstones or peptic ulcers, but if you suffer from those conditions, talk to your doctor before trying it. If you know or suspect that you have lactose or gluten intolerance, the 21-Day Tummy diet can help you figure out exactly what's been troubling your stomach; and if you have celiac disease, it's very easy to modify the diet to shun all sources of gluten. (Notes in Chapters 6 and 7 will alert you to potential sources of gluten.)

What makes *21-Day Tummy* unique is its ability to treat, and sometimes even cure, common digestive disorders.

I'm proud to say that *21-Day Tummy* is the first book I've written to address a specific problem that I've personally dealt with. I'm confident that the 21-Day Tummy diet will help you target the foods that present challenges to your personal digestive system, then show you how to eat in a way that keeps you feeling great—and looking lean—for life.

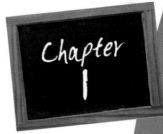

How Our Tummy Troubles Started

It makes sense when you think about it: What you put in your belly affects both how big it gets and how good or bad it feels. And yet I had never made a connection between weight and digestive issues. My eyes started to open when I noticed a few comments that readers had posted online about my last book, *The Digest Diet.* They proudly proclaimed how many pounds they had lost, of course, but they also noted in passing that their stomachs felt better.

So, together with my editors at Reader's Digest, I began to dig and soon uncovered a wealth of research that was being done by scientists—and largely ignored by everyone else. I'll share the highlights of that research with you in the next couple of chapters, but first I want to take a step back to make sure we all understand the magnitude of the problems.

America the Big

The United States is home to the largest population (no pun intended) of obese people in the world.

Consider these statistics from the Centers for Disease Control and Prevention (CDC)[1]:

- Among adults, **33 percent** are overweight and 35 percent are obese.

- Almost three in four men (**74 percent**) and more than 65 percent of women are considered to be overweight or obese.

- Obesity has increased **60 percent** within the past 20 years.

- **One child out of every six** is obese.

- In 2008, medical costs associated with obesity were estimated at **$147 billion;** the medical costs for people who are obese were $1,429 higher than for people of normal weight.

And while the United States may be first in these statistics (a dubious honor indeed!), we're hardly alone. Consider Canada, for instance. Canadian government statistics show that 37 percent of Canadian adults are overweight and 18 percent of adult Canadians are obese.[2] Worldwide, the World Health Organization reports that obesity has nearly doubled since 1980. In 2008, more than 1.4 billion adults over the age of 19 and more than 40 million children under the age of 5 were overweight.[3]

Being overweight or obese increases your risk for heart disease, stroke, type 2 diabetes, and certain types of cancer, all leading causes of preventable death. It puts stress on your joints, makes it harder to breathe, and messes with your digestive system (as we'll learn about in more detail in Chapters 2 and 3).

If you've paid any attention to health news over the past 10 years, you've heard a lot of theories about why rates of overweight and obesity have shot up so much. Fast food and other packaged and processed foods are often fingered as major culprits. One report from the CDC shows that during 2007–2010, adults consumed an average of 11 percent of their total daily calories from fast food and that as the percentage of total daily calories from fast food increased, so did weight.[4]

Portion size is another problem. In the last two decades, portion sizes have ballooned. According to the National

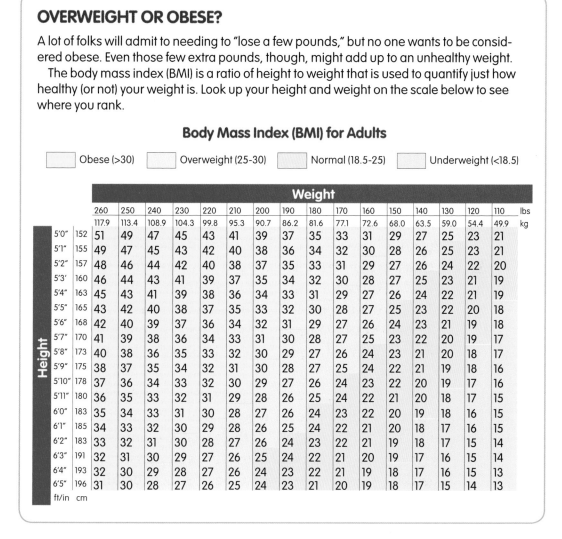

OVERWEIGHT OR OBESE?

A lot of folks will admit to needing to "lose a few pounds," but no one wants to be considered obese. Even those few extra pounds, though, might add up to an unhealthy weight.

The body mass index (BMI) is a ratio of height to weight that is used to quantify just how healthy (or not) your weight is. Look up your height and weight on the scale below to see where you rank.

Body Mass Index (BMI) for Adults

Obese (>30)   Overweight (25-30)   Normal (18.5-25)   Underweight (<18.5)

Height		Weight															
		260	250	240	230	220	210	200	190	180	170	160	150	140	130	120	110	lbs
		117.9	113.4	108.9	104.3	99.8	95.3	90.7	86.2	81.6	77.1	72.6	68.0	63.5	59.0	54.4	49.9	kg
5'0"	152	51	49	47	45	43	41	39	37	35	33	31	29	27	25	23	21
5'1"	155	49	47	45	43	42	40	38	36	34	32	30	28	26	25	23	21
5'2"	157	48	46	44	42	40	38	37	35	33	31	29	27	26	24	22	20
5'3'	160	46	44	43	41	39	37	35	34	32	30	28	27	25	23	21	19
5'4"	163	45	43	41	39	38	36	34	33	31	29	27	26	24	22	21	19
5'5"	165	43	42	40	38	37	35	33	32	30	28	27	25	23	22	20	18
5'6"	168	42	40	39	37	36	34	32	31	29	27	26	24	23	21	19	18
5'7"	170	41	39	38	36	34	33	31	30	28	27	25	23	22	20	19	17
5'8"	173	40	38	36	35	33	32	30	29	27	26	24	23	21	20	18	17
5'9"	175	38	37	35	34	32	31	30	28	27	25	24	22	21	19	18	16
5'10"	178	37	36	34	33	32	30	29	27	26	24	23	22	20	19	17	16
5'11"	180	36	35	33	32	31	29	28	26	25	24	22	21	20	18	17	15
6'0"	183	35	34	33	31	30	28	27	26	24	23	22	20	19	18	16	15
6'1"	185	34	33	32	30	29	28	26	25	24	22	21	20	18	17	16	15
6'2"	183	33	32	31	30	28	27	26	24	23	22	21	19	18	17	15	14
6'3"	191	32	31	30	29	27	26	25	24	22	21	20	19	17	16	15	14
6'4"	193	32	30	29	28	27	26	24	23	22	21	19	18	17	16	15	13
6'5"	196	31	30	28	27	26	25	24	23	21	20	19	18	17	15	14	13
ft/in	cm																

Institutes of Health, 20 years ago, bagels were usually 3 inches and 140 calories. Now? The average bagel today weighs in at 6 inches and 350 calories. Compared to 20 years ago, today's average slice of pizza has 350 more calories, a single soda 165 more calories, and a large popcorn at the movie theater 360 more calories—all because the portions we're typically served are larger now.[5] When people are served more, they eat more. A 2009 article in the *International Journal of Behavioral Nutrition and Physical Activity* showed that when portion sizes were doubled, food intake frequently increased at least 30 percent.[6]

In addition to what and how much we're eating, a big factor in our growing problem (pun intended) is how much we're moving—or rather, how much we're not. Our bodies were designed to be walking (toward food and water), running (away from predators), and reaching (for fruits on trees), not sitting in cars, then staring at a screen for 8 or more hours a day. Sitting too long and not being active is downright dangerous, according to several studies. One 2013 report showed that participants who sat for fewer than 4 hours a day were much less likely to have chronic conditions such as diabetes, heart disease, or high blood pressure than participants who sat for more than 4 hours each day: The longer they sat, the more chronic diseases they suffered from.[7] Even if you're diligent about fitting in fitness, sitting too much can be bad for your waistline and your health, as I learned firsthand after my foot surgery!

Big Bellies Are Not Beautiful

While any kind of excess weight can be problematic, it's especially bad if you carry that weight around your midsection. If you don't know why visceral belly fat is dangerous to your health, here's the Reader's Digest version:

There are two types of belly fat: subcutaneous and visceral. Subcutaneous fat is the stuff we hate to see around our bellies. Sitting just below the skin, it's not pretty, it's not sexy, but it doesn't do much. We can't say the same about visceral fat.

Visceral fat, which we can't even see, surrounds our abdominal organs with a semifluid compound of various types of adipose, or fatty, tissue. It's this compound that really causes our bellies to swell with a serious spare tire. While a number of fancy high-tech ways of measuring visceral fat have been devised, including bioelectrical impedance and magnetic resonance imaging (MRIs), it turns out that the humble tape measure is one of the most accurate. In most people, waist circumference turns out to be a reliable predictor of visceral fat.[8] And, according to a 2008 German study of 360,000 people from nine European countries, having a large waist circumference doubles your risk of death from cancer, stroke, heart disease, and other conditions.[9] Even if you have a normal BMI, you may still have excess visceral fat. Up to

---

HOW TRIM IS YOUR TUMMY?

To measure your waist, use an ultra-flexible tape measure if possible, such as the kind used by seamstresses. If you don't have that, a standard metal tape measure will do.

Start at the top of the hip bone, then bring the tape measure all the way around, level with your belly button. Make sure that it's parallel with the floor and that it's not too tight or too loose. Don't hold your breath. Let your stomach stick out as much as it normally does and, voilà, you have your waist circumference. (You might find it easier to have a spouse or friend help you do this.)

You have a large waist circumference if you are:

- a man with a waist measurement above 40 inches
- a woman with a waist measurement above 35 inches

A large waist circumference puts you at high risk for inflammation and associated illnesses. If your waist circumference is high, it's definitely time for the 21-Day Tummy diet.

40 percent of the population may be "thin on the outside, fat on the inside."[10]

Here's the scariest prospect about belly fat: Research suggests that fat cells are biologically active. Fatty tissue doesn't merely store fat to burn later; fatty tissue is an active metabolic organ, secreting hormones and other substances that contribute to inflammation and promote insulin resistance, the precursor to type 2 diabetes.[11] In a 2012 study in the *Journal of the American Medical Association,* for instance, researchers found that excess visceral fat was associated with an increased risk of type 2 diabetes.[12]

There's another reason why excess visceral fat is so harmful: It's close to the portal vein, which carries blood from your intestines to your liver. The largest organ in the human body, your liver produces bile to carry away waste and break down fat. It also produces cholesterol and special proteins to help carry that fat around the body. When you have too much visceral fat, excess fatty acids in the liver can influence the production of cholesterol in an unhealthy way, increasing blood levels of LDL (bad) cholesterol and lowering levels of HDL (good) cholesterol. These, in turn, are major risk factors for heart disease, type 2 diabetes, stroke, and many other life-threatening issues.

> Even if you have a normal BMI, you may still have excess visceral fat.

Visceral fat has even been linked to cancer risk. A prominent study published in 2013 linked larger waistlines with precancerous colon growths. People with the most visceral fat were more than four times as likely to have precancerous growths compared to those with the least.[13] An earlier study found that women with breast cancer had more visceral fat than women without breast cancer, suggesting a link between cancer and the hormones produced by visceral fat.[14]

In another study conducted by the Fred Hutchinson Cancer Research Center, researchers found that, in a group of people with Barrett's esophagus (a precancerous condition that may be partially caused by heartburn), those with more belly fat were more likely to go on to develop esophageal cancer, an extremely vicious disease—more than 80 percent of patients die within 5 years of diagnosis. This association may be due to the "inflammatory effects of fatty tissue and/or an increase in chronic acid reflux due to the intra-abdominal pressure exerted by extra belly fat," the researchers wrote.[15]

We need a little visceral fat to cushion our organs. Having too much, however, can lead to big problems. I'm on a mission to help Americans reduce visceral fat, and that's a big part of the 21-Day Tummy diet.

Digestive Dictionary

Guess what the difference is between the **digestive tract,** the **gastrointestinal (GI) tract,** and the **gut?** Nothing! These terms are used interchangeably and refer to all the organs needed for digestion, including the stomach and the intestines.

Indigestion Nation

When I started working on this book, I joked with one of my editors that I was going to become the Betty Ford of digestive disorders and destigmatize the issues of constipation, gas, and bloating. But Jamie Lee Curtis and any number of other spokespeople may have beaten me to the punch.

Have you noticed how many ads there are for antacids these days? What about probiotics? Medications and products designed to help you "get regular" or "get out of the bathroom" or otherwise solve your gastrointestinal issues are big business. The global market for medications to treat irritable bowel syndrome (IBS), for example, is expected to rise from $610 million in 2010 to $2.7 billion in 2020.[16] That's a lot of drugs! It doesn't stop with IBS: One-half of American adults have used antacids and 27 percent take two or more per month. Then there are those who use antacids almost daily—nearly 75 percent of total antacid use is by people who take at least six doses per week.[17]

According to the U.S. Department of Health and Human

Services' National Digestive Diseases Information Clearinghouse, 60 million to 70 million Americans are affected by digestive diseases.[18] In addition, more than 20 million Canadians suffer annually from digestive disorders, according to the Canadian Digestive Health Foundation.[19]

Everyone suffers from a little indigestion now and then. It's normal to pass gas up to 20 times a day. And a little queasiness or irregularity from time to time is nothing to worry about. But if you experience nausea, abdominal pain, heartburn, bloating, gas, constipation, or diarrhea on a regular basis, you have a chronic issue.

Kate and I used the nonprofit Rome Foundation's diagnostic criteria as a baseline for defining what's chronic. As a general rule of thumb, if you experience a symptom more than once a week for more than 3 months, then you've joined the ranks of GI sufferers.[20] Severity is also a factor; it's easier to live with mild bloating than stabbing gas pains. (But this is, of course, a very individual thing; if a digestive problem is bothering you enough that you're ready to take action, it's an issue. Check out the Digestion Quiz on page 11 to rate your symptoms.)

You probably already have a theory about what's causing your problem. For you, symptoms arise when you eat something too spicy, too greasy, or too heavy. You may suspect you have a gluten intolerance, or can't digest lactose. Or maybe you just feel uncomfortable after eating too much or too quickly. Of course, soda and other carbonated beverages can cause burping and bloating; acidic foods like oranges and tomatoes may irritate your digestive tract; and too much candy is a sure recipe for a bellyache.

I bet you have your own remedies, too. Perhaps you find comfort in a cup of ginger tea. Maybe you fall back on the BRAT diet (bananas, rice, apples, and plain toast) that is usually prescribed for acute gastroenteritis or food poisoning. If you're really constipated, you might munch on some prunes or drink a fiber supplement. If you suspect you have lactose intolerance, you could avoid dairy or take lactose supplements. If you have heartburn, you may down a little baking soda to neutralize your stomach acid. Or you may look for yogurts with live cultures, digestive teas, or probiotic supplements. And, of course, there are all those pills.

IT'S A FEMALE THING

Women have to deal with all kinds of problems and challenges that men don't. Menstruation, being pregnant, going through labor—and on top of it all, some digestive problems, such as irritable bowel syndrome and gallstones, are more common in women than men, according to the U.S. Department of Health and Human Services Office on Women's Health.

For instance, the menstrual cycle can affect bowel movements. During the second half of a woman's menstrual cycle (immediately after ovulation and before menstruation), women have harder stools. During menstruation, stools are looser and gas increases, according to a study published in *Digestive Diseases and Sciences.*[21]

Pregnant women often get it the worst. Morning sickness, which causes nausea and vomiting, affects up to 80 percent of pregnant women.[22] Pregnancy-related increases in hormones can relax muscles throughout your digestive tract. That means gas doesn't move through, causing excess gas and bloating. It also means stool is slower to pass, causing constipation. Just what a gal needs when she can't see her feet! Those pesky hormones also relax the lower esophageal sphincter separating the esophagus from the stomach. And then, of course, those extra 10 to 20 pounds you're carrying can put pressure on your abdomen, causing acid reflux and heartburn.

If you bring a digestive complaint to your doctor, she'll likely say you need to try something called an elimination diet. This helps you identify your individual trigger foods, foods that trigger a flare-up of your symptoms. Once you've done so, you should avoid those foods for the rest of your life. In the meantime, you'll be advised to stick with bland (read: tasteless) foods, which are thought to be easier to digest. You may also be prescribed various medications to control your symptoms and/or be told to try adding some enzymatic or probiotic supplements. Sounds pretty grim, doesn't it? No wonder so many of us decide it's better to just live with discomfort!

But while these theories and remedies have some merit, most of them only address the symptoms you are experiencing, not their causes. In order to get more lasting relief, you need to tackle the problems underlying all your digestive woes. That's exactly what the 21-Day Tummy diet does. Like an elimination diet, it cuts out potential trigger foods—including ones you've never heard about before—to calm your belly quickly and get you symptom-free. But whereas the elimination diet is like a firehose that flushes everything out of your system, the 21-Day Tummy plan is a water pick that strategically cleanses, removing just the troublesome stuff and leaving you plenty of delicious and nutritious food to eat. In fact, the plan actually adds nutrients, such as magnesium and MUFAs, which have been shown to help shrink and soothe your belly at the same time. And while the elimination diet isn't sustainable (plain bread and rice is not only boring, it doesn't give you varied enough nutrition), you'll find that you can happily and healthfully follow the 21-Day Tummy way of eating for life.

The Weight-Digestion Link

There's a sordid relationship between digestive problems and extra weight. Both can lead to serious illness, and the factors that create extra weight—our unbalanced gut flora and chronic inflammation—often make digestion difficult. I imagine these partners in crime walking hand in hand down an alleyway, laughing maniacally at my unwanted 10 pounds and my worsening constipation. The 21-Day Tummy plan tackles these tummy tormentors with a one-two punch.

(continued on page 14)

Rate Your DQ

Before we learn more about digestion, let's find out how yours is doing. Maybe you feel bloated, get acid reflux, or become crampy and gaseous after eating. These observations are important, but let's go a step further and quantify. Too often, many of us think our digestive symptoms are normal, so we just live with the discomfort. For years, I accepted my own symptoms as just a normal part of being me. As the years went by and my issues worsened, I knew it was time for change. The following quiz is very quick and will help you rate your digestion. If you experience severe digestive problems (such as intense pain or passing blood or mucus, which could be the sign of several serious illnesses), see your doctor!

The Digestion Quiz

1. Do you have heartburn more than once a month? If so, assign one point.

2. Do you have heartburn once a week or more? If so, assign one point.

3. Do you have a bowel movement every day? If so, assign zero points.

4. Do you have a bowel movement fewer than five times a week? If so, assign one point.

5. Do you have loose stools or diarrhea about once a week? If so, assign one point.

6. Do you have loose stools or diarrhea almost every day? If so, assign one point.

7. Are your stools hard and dry more than once a month? If so, assign one point.

8. Are your stools hard and dry once a week or more? If so, assign one point.

9. Do you feel bloated (exclude menstrual bloat) more than twice a month? If so, assign one point.

10. Do you feel bloated (exclude menstrual bloat) more than once a week? If so, assign one point.

11. Do you experience stomach pain (exclude menstrual pain) more than once a month? If so, assign one point.

12. Do you experience stomach pain (exclude menstrual pain) more than once a week? If so, assign one point.

13. At least 75 percent of the time, are your stools generally like the following: in one piece, snakelike, and easy to pass? If so, assign zero points.

14. Do you experience foul-smelling gas on most days (think rotten-egg caliber)? If so, assign one point.

15. Do you experience an increase in gas as the day progresses? If so, assign one point.

SCORE: Add up all your points. The key is below.

*0–4 points: Congratulations! Your digestion seems to be in good working order. There may be room for improvement, but overall, your GI tract is in decent to great shape. You can still benefit from the 21-Day Tummy diet though, to help keep your digestion humming along and to trim belly inches.

*5–8 points: Your digestion needs a little help. Sometimes it's on the right track and you feel healthy, and sometimes you have problems that cause discomfort or embarrassment. These smallish upsets can lead to bigger problems down the road if you don't deal with them now. Time for the 21-Day Tummy diet!

*9–15 points: Ouch! Your digestion is hurting, which means you are, too. You found the 21-Day Tummy diet just in time. This plan will help you feel better fast—and will help you flatten your belly.

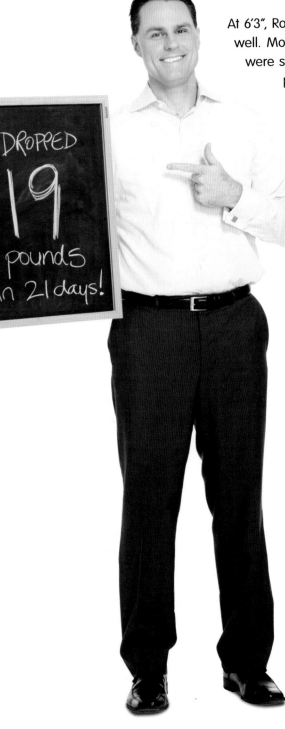

At 6'3", Rob is tall enough to carry his weight well. Most of his colleagues (me included!) were surprised to learn that he had extra pounds to lose—but at 233 pounds, his BMI put him on the high end of the "overweight" category. And he was feeling it. He was usually exhausted by day's end, and the bursitis pain in his right shoulder was flaring up more frequently.

Plus, he had constant, severe heartburn. He had been relying on daily prescription medication to control the symptoms and, previously, when he had tried to wean him-

No more daily heartburn medication!

self off of it, as soon as he skipped a dose, he felt a lot of discomfort. But on day 1 of the 21-Day Tummy diet, "I stopped taking the medication, and I did not need it once. My acid reflux is completely gone." Amazing!

Rob almost didn't try the diet. Because he had several business trips plus a vacation scheduled during the 21-day trial, he wasn't sure he would be able to follow the plan. But he found it easy to find belly-friendly foods when eating out—and once he started seeing results, it was easy to avoid the temptations offered by his dining companions!

Rob's goal had been to "start the journey of losing 15 pounds," but he didn't necessarily expect to do it all in 21 days. Instead, he blew away his expectations, dropping a whopping 19 pounds—that's almost a pound a day! "To know that I lost even more than I wanted. . . . I just simply feel better about myself. This plan is giving me more confidence. I have more stamina and less exhaustion by day's end. I'm sleeping better as well.

"Compared to other diets, the weight loss of the 21-Day Tummy diet was much quicker. Other plans took 3 or 4 months to accomplish what I did here in 3 weeks. I've been able to kick the 'habit' of eating just to eat, and now I eat when I'm truly hungry—and choose satisfying foods."

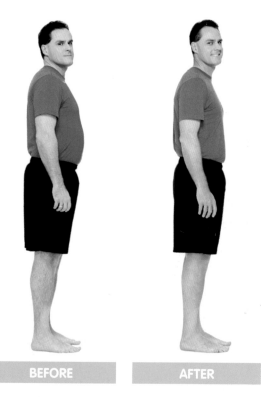

| BEFORE | AFTER |

Rob McMahon

Age 42

Lost 19 POUNDS and 2½ BELLY INCHES in 21 days!

Proudest accomplishments: Dropped more than his goal weight; stopped taking heartburn medication completely!

Favorite recipes: Ginger and Tomato Flank Steak; Tomato Lime Quinoa Salad

(continued from page 10)

The Role of Gut Bacteria

Did you know that the human body can carry up to 6 pounds of bacteria?[24] This is not a problem. In fact, these micro-organisms turn out to be pretty useful to have around. "Good" bacteria keep the digestive system healthy by performing several essential functions.

They provide a physical barrier by coating the digestive tract, and they convert food into substances that nourish the lining of the gut. They also produce enzymes that break down food and manufacture nutrients, including vitamin K and several B vitamins. Some, such as *Lactobacillus acidophilus*, help our bodies absorb minerals such as calcium and magnesium;[25] others, such as *Streptococcus thermophiles* and *Bifidobacterium bifidum*, may protect against toxic substances like mercury.[26] Beneficial gut microbiota may even maintain the immune system's defenses against disease. For example, certain bacteria such as *Bifidobacterium infantis* can reduce the symptoms of IBS, such as diarrhea.[27]

> **KNOWLEDGE NIBBLES**
> Where doctors had previously isolated only a few hundred bacterial species from the body, researchers now calculate that more than 10,000 microbial species occupy the human ecosystem.[23]

An imbalance of bacteria in our gastrointestinal tract, though, leads to weight gain and a host of digestive ills, and leaves you vulnerable to disease. If you have too few good bacteria, of course, you'll lose out on the benefits they provide. If you have too many "bad" bacteria, some may directly cause digestive upsets such as colitis or even increase the tumor growth rate in some cancers.[28] Imbalanced gut flora can also make constipation, diarrhea, gas, bloating, and IBS worse. It's not that certain types of bacteria automatically cause certain illnesses; it's all about the balance versus imbalance of a great many types of bacteria.[29] The total number of bacteria in our GI system and exactly where in our digestive tract they live can also make a difference. Yes, it's complicated!

The Human Microbiome Project has attempted to sort the good from the bad and has proven so far that bacteria are indeed integral to health and digestion. Hundreds of scientists from 80 universities and research institutions have spent the last five years genetically mapping 81 to 99 percent of our normal bacterial makeup and have found strong links between bad bacteria and extra weight.

"Lean and obese people have markedly different communities [of bacteria] in the gut," said Rob Knight, PhD, associate professor at the BioFrontiers Institute at the University of Colorado–Boulder. "We don't know if microbes contribute to weight gain or if they change when people become obese." In short, overweight people have different bacteria in their guts than thin people have, and those differences may make them fatter.

In a 2009 article examining the link between weight and gut flora, researchers wrote: "Studies demonstrate that certain mixes of gut microbiota may protect or predispose the host to obesity [by] increasing dietary energy harvest, promoting fat deposition, and triggering systemic inflammation."[30] I don't think too many of us are hoping for more fat to be deposited anywhere on our bodies. And while it might sound good to increase your "dietary energy harvest," I'm

PROBIOTICS: A PRIMER

The term probiotics refers to microbes such as bacteria or yeast that "promote life" by providing healthful benefits to their host—that would be us. Probiotics can be found in some fermented foods. Not all fermented foods, though, contain probiotics. And some that do also contain other substances that can bother your belly (see box on page 43 for more details). The 21-Day Tummy eating plan features Greek yogurt, one of the best tummy-friendly food sources of probiotics, and steers clear of other potentially problematic probiotic-containing foods.

Probiotics can also commonly be found as supplements in health food stores, either as capsules, powders, or liquids. We don't recommend adding probiotic supplements during the 21-Day Tummy diet because we want to make sure the plan's healing foods are doing their work. (If you are already taking probiotics and find they are helpful, then by all means continue using them.) After your first 21 days, if you're still experiencing some digestive issues, you can try some probiotic supplements. Look for ones labeled "enteric coated"; these are acid and enzyme resistant so that they can travel through your stomach safely to your intestines. Follow dosing instructions to make sure you get enough to provide a benefit.

sure you'll change your tune when you realize that that means that your bacteria are getting more calories out of your food, contributing to weight gain.

A 2013 study demonstrated how this can happen. Researchers at Cedars-Sinai used breath analysis to determine what microorganisms, and in what amount, the participants had in their guts. It turns out that your breath can tell a lot more than whether you forgot to brush your teeth. The subjects either had normal breath content, higher concentrations of methane, higher levels of hydrogen, or higher levels of both gases. Of the 792 subjects, those who tested positive for high concentrations of both methane and hydrogen had significantly higher body mass indexes and higher percentages of body fat.[31]

Gut bacteria could harvest more calories from your food, leading to weight gain.

A microorganism called *Methanobrevibacter smithii* produces the majority of a person's methane, scavenging hydrogen from other microbes and using it to manufacture the gas. Researchers believe that the interaction of those organisms helps neighboring hydrogen-producing bacteria extract nutrients from food more efficiently.

"Essentially, [this] could allow a person to harvest more calories from their food," said lead author Ruchi Mathur. So when *M. smithii* becomes overabundant, people are more likely to gain weight. "This is the first large-scale human study to show an association between gas production and body weight—and this could prove to be another important factor in understanding one of the many causes of obesity." (Adding insult to injury, *M. smithii* may also cause constipation![32])

Gut bacteria may also contribute to inflammation, a factor in obesity and many other chronic diseases. In a study that examined more than 300 people, subjects who had high levels of inflammatory markers had the lowest levels of good bacteria, suggesting that good bacteria could protect against an out-of-control inflammatory response.[33]

In addition to digestive discord and extra weight, imbalances in our gut flora have been implicated in diseases ranging from autism and allergies to high blood pressure and heart disease. According to a 2013 study from Johns Hopkins University and Yale University, a specialized receptor in our blood vessels senses small molecules created by our gut bacteria when we eat. The receptor responds to those molecules by increasing blood pressure. After we finish eating, the gut microbes give off a signal that causes the receptors to decrease blood pressure. Thus, our gut bacteria help regulate blood pressure.[34] Meanwhile, a series of studies conducted at the Cleveland Clinic demonstrated that when gut bacteria break down lecithin and carnitine—substances found in meat, egg, and dairy foods—it leads to the creation of a substance that encourages fatty plaque deposits to form in your arteries. Known as atherosclerosis, this is a major risk factor for heart disease.[35, 36]

Gut bacteria can even change your brain function, according to a 2013 study. Researchers took functional magnetic resonance imaging (fMRI) scans of healthy women's brains while they were at rest and while they were viewing pictures of people with angry or frightened faces. In both instances, they saw marked differences between women who were given probiotic yogurt to eat daily and those who weren't.[37] The researchers were surprised to find that the brain effects could be seen in many areas, including those involved in sensory processing and not merely those associated with emotion, said Dr. Kirsten Tillisch, an associate professor of medicine at UCLA's David Geffen School of Medicine and lead author of the study. "Our findings indicate that some of the contents of yogurt may actually change the way our brain responds to the environment. When we consider the implications of this work, the old sayings 'you are what you eat' and 'gut feelings' take on new meaning."

Why is gut flora so closely tied to many different illnesses? The reason is our immune system. Gut microbes help develop and maintain the immune system; they also help absorb nutrients from our food that aid our immune function. When our

(continued on page 19)

Adrienne Farr

Before learning about the 21-Day Tummy plan, Adrienne had already lost more than 60 pounds on the Digest Diet. So she knew a thing or two about how to trim her waistline! But her weight loss had slowed, and she was experiencing stomach pain, bloating, and nausea 3 or 4 days a week. On the 21-Day Tummy plan, she dropped 6½ pounds and 3 inches from her waist, and her digestive symptoms almost completely disappeared!

Q: What surprised you about this diet?

A: I had no idea that onions and garlic cause problems with your digestive tract if you're sensitive to them. I've always heard that both of those things were good and healthy so that was very, very shocking to me. I figure it must be true because I haven't eaten any of those [Belly Bully] foods in three weeks and my digestion issues are so much better and my belly doesn't feel bloated.

Q: What was one of your favorite parts of this diet?

A: It's not all about the weight. It's about how you feel and it's about taking care of your digestion. I had been feeling discouraged about how little weight I was losing so it was a breakthrough when I realized that it had been a long time since I'd had a cramp or felt bloated.

Q: What did you think of the recipes?

A: I loved them. They weren't that hard, either. I feel like I was in and out of the kitchen a lot of times in like, a half an hour. The Lemony Salmon, Potato, and Dill Bake was my favorite; I made that for my mother, who usually eats a lot of unhealthy stuff like macaroni and cheese, and she loved it.

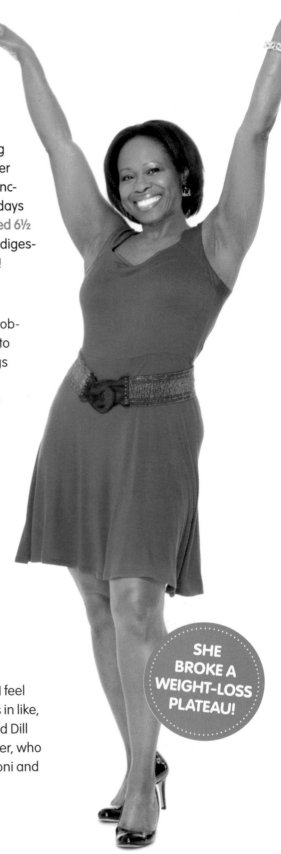

SHE BROKE A WEIGHT-LOSS PLATEAU!

(continued from page 17)

gut flora is out of whack, so is our immune system, and we are left vulnerable to a dizzying array of illnesses.[38] One of the hallmarks of an immune system gone awry? Chronic inflammation.

The Role of Inflammation

Inflammation is our body's response to injury. We usually think of it as an external thing. When we catch our finger in the door, it swells up. When a bug bites us, we get a red itchy rash. The inflammatory response acts as a first line of defense for the immune system, a bodyguard at the ready. Although inflammation may not be pleasant, it's necessary to the healing process and helps repair damaged tissue.

Inflammation also happens on a cellular level. Imagine the cells in your body swelling up and you understand how inflammation can make you fat. But it's not that simple. Cellular inflammation sets off a complex chemical chain reaction inside your body that can lead to a wide range of problems—including digestive disorders and excess weight—if it becomes chronic.

> When your immune system overreacts, leading to chronic inflammation, you're very likely to feel it in your tummy.

It's in your gut that your immune system is most likely to kick into high gear; after all, that's the one place where you are regularly introducing foreign substances—i.e., food—into your body. Our gut houses 70 percent of our immune function.[39] This is helpful for fending off harmful viruses, bacteria, and other pathogens that may be lurking in your food. But it also means that when your immune system overreacts, leading to chronic inflammation, you're very likely to feel it in your tummy.

Inflammatory bowel disease (IBD) is, just as it sounds, a condition that occurs when you have a chronically inflamed digestive tract. Crohn's disease and ulcerative colitis are the most common types of IBD and differ primarily in the location of the inflammation; Crohn's can affect any part of the GI tract, while colitis appears in the colon and rectum. Symptoms can include abdominal pain and cramping, diarrhea, and bloody stools. Chronic inflammation can also contribute to other digestive disorders, such as gallbladder disease and pancreatitis, as well as to milder but still bothersome symptoms such as uncomfortable gas, bloating, or constipation.

There's a close relationship between gut flora, inflammation, excess weight, and illness.

IBD can sometimes cause weight loss because your inflamed digestive tract is not able to do its job of extracting nutrition from food. (Since this can also lead to malnutrition and other complications, though, I wouldn't recommend it as a way to drop the pounds!) Not all inflammation in the digestive tract is classed as IBD, though. Food allergies, which occur when your immune system mistakes a food for an invader, also set off an inflammatory response, as do low-grade bacterial or viral infections.

To combat this inflammation, your body naturally produces anti-inflammatory chemicals. These chemicals interfere with the function of the hormone leptin. When leptin is working properly, it signals your brain to stop eating as soon as your fat stores are full. But when inflammation becomes chronic, your brain no longer gets the message. Even though you've consumed enough to fuel your body, you still feel hungry, so you overeat and gain weight. This condition is called leptin resistance, and it usually comes hand in hand with excess body fat.[40] In one long-running study of more than 6,000 men, those who had elevated levels of 5 different inflammatory markers all gained weight later in life.[41] In short, inflammation made them fat.

Because inflammation can happen anywhere in your body, it's linked to a wide range of diseases, not just digestive issues and extra weight. Chronic inflammation can cause arthritis (when your joints are inflamed), heart disease and stroke (when inflammation in blood vessels cause atherosclerosis or clots), or type 2 diabetes (when leptin resistance leads to insulin resistance and then to diabetes). Chronic inflammation may even contribute to some cancers. First, it damages the immune functions that fight off infections that set the stage for some cancers. Then, it produces substances that increase the risk of DNA mutations that cause cells to become cancerous. Finally, inflammation can kill healthy cells, paving the way for tumor growth.[42]

You'll see that there's a lot of overlap between the health problems associated with gut flora imbalances and those associated with inflammation. That's because there's a close relationship between gut flora, inflammation, excess weight, and illness.

***

Now that we've uncovered the real underlying causes of your tummy troubles—an imbalance in your gut flora and chronic inflammation—let's learn what really goes on in your gut.

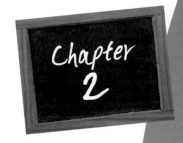

Belly Basics:
What Works,
What's Wrong

Most of us don't give much thought to digestion because it seems so easy: Chew, swallow, wait. But this enormously complicated process taxes the body, even when everything is working well. It takes a great deal of energy to break down food. When we give our bodies the wrong types of food or too much food, when we are stressed out and ill rested, we make digestion even harder. Using more energy might sound like a good way to burn more calories. But those calories burned aren't worth the damage that we do to our systems when we make the digestive tract and its associated organs work too hard.

An almost unfathomably complex series of events takes place from the time food goes in your body until the time it goes out. It helped me understand the 21-Day Tummy plan to learn precisely how digestion works.

Good Digestion:
What You're Aiming For

Our digestive system consists of organs that are connected to a long tube, about 30 feet in length, that stretches from the mouth to the anus. The tube changes considerably along the way (the esophagus is far different from the small intestine), but the purpose is similar at every stretch: to propel, break down, and extract nutrients from food. Undulating muscles lining the GI tract help move food through.

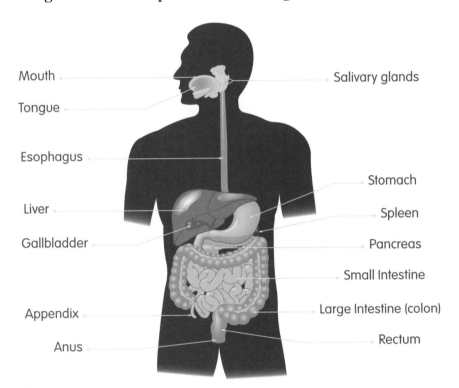

Mouth

Tongue

Esophagus

Liver

Gallbladder

Appendix

Anus

Salivary glands

Stomach

Spleen

Pancreas

Small Intestine

Large Intestine (colon)

Rectum

The journey starts at the mouth. We chew, which changes the shape of the food and combines it with saliva. Chewing increases the surface area of food, which gives the enzymes in your saliva more access to its nutrients. Some research also suggests that chewing signals the rest of the body to begin the digestion process. The more you chew, the more the food circulates through your mouth, and that increases the amount and degree to which taste receptors have access to it. When taste receptors detect food, the stomach begins producing the acid that is so important to digestion. Finally, the moisture of saliva helps the food pass down our esophagus, which happens when we swallow.

Chewing and swallowing are voluntary, but once we swallow, our bodies take over in a dizzying process of involuntary actions.

The esophagus connects the throat to the stomach, which has three main roles. First, it stores food we swallow. Then, it mixes the solid parts of the food, along with any liquid we've consumed, with digestive juices (also called gastric juices) that the stomach produces. Finally, it empties the resulting contents, called chyme, into the small intestine.

The small intestine is where most of the digestive process takes place. While powerful muscles move the mixture through this 20-foot-long tube, the food continues to mix with digestive juices from the pancreas and liver and gets broken down to even smaller pieces. At the same time, the walls of the small intestine absorb nutrients from that food and transport them through the body. This, of course, is the point of eating; ideally, we eat to feed the right nutrition to our various body parts so they function best. After the nutrients are absorbed from our food, what's left is everything we couldn't digest— mostly fiber and water.

THE SLIMMING WAY TO CHEW

It takes about 20 minutes for your gut to tell your brain that it's full, so the slower you eat, the less you will have consumed before you get that "Stop, I'm full!" message.

Plus, you burn calories when you chew. According to a study of 450 women in Japan, those who ate foods that required the most chewing shaved more than an inch from their bellies compared to those who ate the softest foods.[1] And taking time to chew your food is essential for proper digestion, breaking food into small enough pieces for the rest of your GI tract to handle and signaling your stomach to begin producing acid.

How long should you chew a bite of food? Answers vary, but research from Iowa State University, presented at the Experimental Biology 2012 Conference in San Diego, found that chewing food at least 40 times is not only good for digestion, but also helps people eat less.[2] If you feel foolish counting, try just chewing until you can no longer tell what the food was by its texture. That's obviously easier to do with mashed potatoes than with raw carrots, but that just means the raw carrots should be chewed more. Consider chewing as the heavy lifting of digestion. Chomp away!

The small intestine pushes this lovely mix into the large intestine, also called the colon. The colon's most important job is to remove water from the food that passes through it. When food moves through too quickly, the colon might not remove enough water, causing diarrhea. When food moves through too slowly, then too much water is removed, resulting in constipation.

The colon is also where most of our gut bacteria live. The acid, bile, and pancreatic juices in the stomach and small intestine make it difficult for bacteria to thrive, though a few hardy species do. But it's in the large intestine where most of them flourish, feasting on all the food we couldn't digest and helping us to extract even more nutrition from it. Our gut flora does so much, in fact, that it can be considered an extra digestive organ.[3]

The last place in the digestive system, the rectum is the official home of the feces—until, that is, a bowel movement occurs. That last great push of undulations expels the feces out of our body, and digestion is complete.

The Digestive Juice Bar

The mucosa that lines our gastrointestinal tract contains incredibly small glands that produce enzyme-rich digestive juices. Substances that start and/or speed up chemical reactions, these enzymes break food down into the nutrients your body needs to function—carbohydrates split into sugars, protein into amino acids, and fats into fatty acids.

Salivary glands in your mouth produce saliva (salivary: saliva—the logic!), and saliva contains enzymes that divide starch and fat into smaller molecules. Next, the digestive glands of your stomach lining produce hydrochloric acid (HCL). HCL activates the enzyme pepsin, which breaks down protein. HCL also kills potentially dangerous pathogens in our food. Now, "acid" may not sound like a comfortable item to have in the body, but actually it's perfectly safe. You're shielded from this acid (unless you have ulcers) because of a thick layer of mucus that protects your stomach tissue.

Next, your stomach empties the sugars, amino acids, and fatty acids from your food into the small intestine. Here, enzymes in the walls of the small intestine split the sugars and amino acids into even smaller pieces, while digestive juices from the pancreas help to break down all kinds of nutrients. Also, when you start eating, your gallbladder squeezes bile (which, confusingly, is actually produced by the liver) into the intestines where it helps dissolve fat. As you can see when you try to wash grease off dishes, dissolving fat is no easy feat. Bile acts like dishwashing liquid, breaking the remaining fatty acids into digestible pieces.

The digestive juice bar stops around this point—there are no enzymes in the large intestine. Some food still gets digested here, though, thanks to our gut flora; some bacteria help us break down food and absorb the nutrients from them.

As you can see, each type of food requires different enzymes to help our body digest it. If we don't have the appropriate

THE COLORFUL FACES OF FECES

Normal, healthy stool is a medium shade of brown. If it turns other colors, it can be a sign of a problem. Here's a rundown of some of the shades to watch out for:

COLOR	POTENTIAL CAUSES
Red	Beets; food dye; internal bleeding; hemorrhoids
Yellow	Too much fat; gallbladder dysfunction; pancreatic enzyme insufficiency
Black	Internal bleeding; excess iron consumption; a meat-heavy diet; Pepto-Bismol
White	Improper fat absorption; pancreatitis and pancreatic cancer; barium (used for x-rays); inflammation; excess mucous; IBS
Clay colored	Liver disease; antacids that contain aluminum hydroxide (such as Maalox, Mylanta); some vitamins and supplements (such as vitamin A); bismuth subsalicylate (such as Kaopectate, Pepto-Bismol) and other anti-diarrheal drugs

enzymes, then we can't digest that food properly and it becomes food for our gut bacteria, which can cause gas and bloating. excess gas, bloating, and other symptoms. If you know that you are deficient in a specific enzyme, such as lactase, taking supplemental digestive enzymes can help. Other enzymes that can help are alpha-galactosidase (the active ingredient in Beano), which breaks down oligosaccharides in beans, and lipases, which help digest fat.

However, because so many different factors can cause GI symptoms, many people misdiagnose themselves. If you notice that your tummy grumbles every time you have pizza, for instance, you might assume that you are lactose intolerant. But it's possible that the problem is actually the fructans, a type of fiber, in the pizza crust (see box on page 29). So you might get some benefit from the placebo effect when you take lactase supplements, but you would still have some symptoms. Plus, while lactase supplements do help digest lactose, they might not get to all the lactose in your food (especially if your digestive system works fast and speeds the lactose through).

On the 21-Day Tummy plan, we want to make sure we calm your tummy completely. You'll remove all potentially problematic foods for these three weeks so you won't need supplemental digestive enzymes during this time. Then you'll test each one to learn what's *really* bothering your belly. Once you've figured that out, you'll know whether a supplemental digestive enzyme would help you and if so, which one.

The Speed of Digestion

Ever notice how the effects of eating just one big meal can stay with you for days? While it usually takes about 6 to 8 hours for food to pass through the stomach and small intestine, it can take up to 3 days to completely digest a meal!

A number of things affect how fast or slow your digestive system works. First, different foods break down at different rates. In general, carbohydrates move through the system the fastest, protein stays longer, and fats can really linger.[5]

One exception is fiber. A type of carbohydrate found in many fruits, vegetables, and grains, fiber is not absorbed or digested by the body; basically, what goes in, comes out. Fiber can be soluble (meaning, it's dissolvable in water) or insoluble (meaning, it's not). Soluble fiber is often found in the flesh of fruits and vegetables while insoluble fiber is in the skin.

Soluble fiber combines with water during digestion, turns into a gel, and slows down the digestive process. Because it stays in your system for a little while, it helps you feel full longer, so you eat less. Insoluble fiber creates bulk, and that bulk helps us move stool more easily. It can also move harmful carcinogens through the digestive tract and out of our bodies—yay! Insoluble fiber increases regularity and decreases constipation and sluggishness. That's what I needed!

In addition, exercise and stress can affect how quickly the muscles of your small intestine move food through your system. Interestingly, both of these factors can either speed up or slow down muscle contractions,

TUMMY TWISTER OR TAMER? Prebiotics

Prebiotics are non-digestible food components—fibers—that feed gut microbes. These are helpful for many people. But for people who are sensitive to them, certain prebiotics may contribute to uncomfortable gas or bloating. (Note that while all prebiotics are fibers, not all fibers are prebiotics.)

The prebiotics best studied are fructans and galacto-oligosaccharides (GOS). Fructans in particular are known to enhance bifidobacteria, which has been linked with a decreased risk of colon cancer.[6] Two small studies suggest that some types of fructans and GOS may help you feel full longer after eating.[7, 8] But as you'll learn, fructans and GOS are also FODMAPs, rapidly fermentable carbohydrates that can cause digestive upset.

The 21-Day Tummy diet reduces FODMAPs to eliminate the possibility of excess gas and other GI symptoms. But after you finish the 21-day plan, we'll show you how to figure out which prebiotics are a problem for you and which are helpful.

depending on the individual and the situation. For example, running and other aerobic exercises usually speed up muscle contractions, while yoga may slow them down.[9] Stress may give some people the runs but constipate others.

Finally, microbes that produce methane may make our large intestine sluggish while hydrogen-producing gut flora have been shown to help speed it up.[10]

How Digestion Can Go Wrong

Now that you see what a healthy digestion process looks like, it's easy to imagine how it can go wrong. It's all necessary—the juices, enzymes, organs, bacteria, muscles—and a problem anywhere along the line can lead to some serious tummy aches.

As I described in the last chapter, chronic inflammation and an imbalance in your gut flora are key causes of both excess weight and common digestive issues. So what causes the imbalance and the inflammation?

The Microbial Balancing Act

We are not born with bacteria in our guts. But as soon as we leave the shelter of our mother's womb, we come into contact with hundreds of thousands of micro-organisms. Some of them take up residence in our digestive tract and start to multiply. As I mentioned in the last chapter, many of these microbes prove to be helpful houseguests, so we happily coexist with them, a condition called symbiosis. We remain in symbiosis as long as we have more good bacteria than bad bacteria in our microbiome. When our bacterial population thins out, or when the bad bacteria start to outweigh the good, this imbalance is called dysbiosis.

> We remain in symbiosis as long as we have more good bacteria than bad bacteria in our microbiome.

Friendly flora make essential nutrients, protect against toxins, and strengthen your immunity. Unfriendly microbes cause inflammation, weight gain, and ill health. What changes the balance between our good and bad gut bacteria?

Infections by unfriendly bacteria, viruses, or parasites can overwhelm beneficial bacteria.

Antibiotics designed to kill bad bacteria can also kill good ones.

Stress can reduce the numbers of helpful Bacteroides and increase the relative abundance of disease-causing Clostridium, according to a 2011 study from Ohio State University.[11]

Pregnancy can impact the microbiome. Researchers at Cornell University recently discovered that the microbiota of pregnant women resembled that of people at risk for diabetes. Both populations have a high amount of Proteobacteria and Actinobacteria, which have been associated with inflammation.[12] (But don't worry, ladies! The study noted that these changes did not affect mothers' health.) The researchers speculated that the changes in gut bacteria balance may help pregnant women gain weight when they need to.

Changes in weight can change the balance of gut flora, for good or bad. A Washington University School of Medicine study showed that people who lost weight (as a result of two different types of low-calorie diets) saw an increase in the amount of their beneficial bacteria Bacteroidetes.[13] As we saw in Chapter 1, *Methanobrevibacter smithii* can contribute to weight gain, so clearly there's a two-way relationship between our weight and our gut flora.

Diet also changes how many and what types of bacteria live in your gut. In a recent University of Pennsylvania study, 10 people were sequestered so what they ate could be tightly

> ## HOW ANTIBIOTICS WREAK HAVOC
>
> Antibiotics are, by definition, substances that kill bacteria. If you are prescribed antibiotics, take them exactly as your doctor instructs. Some people take antibiotics until they feel better, then ignore the rest of the bottle. This is a great way to breed a monster infection. That's right: Taking antibiotics and then stopping them prematurely can make the original infection much worse.
>
> In addition to killing the bad bacteria that has made you sick, antibiotics will also kill your healthy bacteria. The loss of these healthy bacteria can wreak havoc on digestion. So once you've finished a course of antibiotics, consider taking a probiotic to replace the good bacteria.

(continued on page 33)

Jaimie Hoffman

Before *21-Day Tummy,* Jaimie says, her stomach was a "mess." Not only did she have occasional diarrhea and constipation, but after she ate, she regularly experienced bloating and gas pain. By the end of the day, she reported, "I'm almost an entire size larger in pants due to my belly." With the 21-Day Tummy plan, though, her GI symptoms had all disappeared. As an added bonus, Jaimie lost 3 pounds and almost 2 inches from her waist.

Q: What surprised you about the diet?

A: I feel like my clothes fit me a different way (even when I've been at this same size). This might be because my stomach is not bloated. And my wedding ring fits now! Because my fingers would swell, I haven't been able to wear my ring in a long time. I'm looking and feeling good . . . I'm in a great mood because of this diet!

Q: How did the diet compare to others you've tried?

A: I've tried just restricting calories in the past, but as I'm getting older, it's just not working for me. I used to work out about four to five times a week without seeing any difference in my size or shape. With this plan, I feel good in my belly—so much so I didn't "notice" it anymore!

Q: What have you learned from the 21-Day Tummy diet?

A: I have learned that you are what you eat. If you are eating things that aren't good for you, your body produces things that aren't good for you—so if you balance it out, then your body will be balanced. Also, it now seems pretty clear that I have a gluten intolerance so I'm going to give gluten-free living a try!

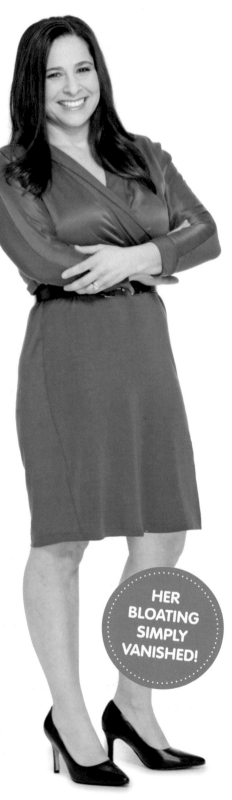

HER BLOATING SIMPLY VANISHED!

(continued from page 31)

controlled. Within 24 hours, researchers saw marked changes in the composition of their gut microbiota.[14] Interestingly, different bacteria were affected in each person, indicating that the effects of what you eat vary in each individual.

New research has identified specific foods that influence gut flora. Korean researchers fed mice a high-fat diet for 8 weeks and found that they grew more obesity-related Firmicutes bacteria and fewer helpful Bacteroides bacteria. Inflammation in their large intestines also surged.[15] According to another study, mice who got 37 percent of their calories from saturated fat (about the same proportion as the standard American diet), had a much higher percentage of *Bilophila wadsworthia,* a harmful microbe associated with inflammatory bowel disease, than mice who ate mostly unsaturated fats.[16]

In addition to saturated fats, rapidly fermentable carbohydrates called FODMAPs promote the growth of gut flora. Indeed, as I'll explain in a little more detail later in this chapter, FODMAPs are a prime source of food for your bacteria, so the more FODMAPs you eat, the more bacteria you have. This can lead to gas and bloating, depending on which FODMAPs you eat and which you're sensitive to.

Inflammation and Imbalance: A Vicious Cycle

Inflammation, as you'll recall from Chapter 1, is your immune system's response to outside threats. Normally, when your body detects a potential problem—say, a viral infection—it releases inflammatory chemicals to isolate and destroy the virus; then, when it senses that the problem has been resolved, your immune system releases anti-inflammatory chemicals to turn off the inflammatory response.

If the infection isn't eradicated, though, or if it recurs frequently, then inflammation becomes chronic. Chronic inflammation can also occur when your immune system makes a mistake, attacking innocent substances like food (as in food allergies) or missing the cues that the threats are not real (as in chronic stress). What might contribute to chronic inflammation?

Repeated infections by unfriendly bacteria, viruses, or parasites can keep triggering a damaging inflammatory response.

Continued exposure to environmental toxins like mercury, lead, or tobacco also fits the definition of a repeated outside threat.

Chronic stress is another common culprit. Stress raises levels of the hormone cortisol, which normally helps to turn off the inflammatory response. In a pair of Carnegie Mellon University studies, healthy adults were exposed to a cold virus. Those who experienced more stress were less able to shut down their inflammatory response. Their bodies had become desensitized to cortisol, so their immune cells ignored its messages to stop inflammation. These subjects produced more cytokines, the chemical messengers in your cells that trigger inflammation, and were more likely to develop cold symptoms.[17]

Another issue with those elevated cortisol levels? They also interfere with the effectiveness of insulin, the hormone that's responsible for telling cells to collect sugar from your bloodstream. That means sugar doesn't get to the cells that need it, so those cells send out signals to the brain saying that they're starving. The brain then sends out hormones, including leptin, that cause you to

THE HEAVY EFFECTS OF SLEEP DEPRIVATION

Lack of sleep interferes with the normal workings of your hunger hormones, causing cravings for high-calorie comfort foods. After all, if you're not well-rested, you need energy from some other source—and because they are so rapidly digested, sugary and carb-heavy foods give you the quickest hit. Even worse, it turns out that these hormonal changes lead our body to deposit the extra weight we gain from these foods right where we want it least—around our belly.[18]

Food and sleep are linked in another interesting way. According to a study from the University of Pennsylvania, people who sleep 7 to 8 hours each night eat a greater variety of foods than people who sleep less.[19] It seems a varied diet that spans the food groups, like the 21-Day Tummy meal plan, is not only the spice of life but also essential to a good night's sleep.

crave sweets and fatty foods, overeat them, and gain weight.

Weight gain, in turn, leads to more inflammation. Elevated cortisol leads to an increase in visceral fat as it relocates fat from your bloodstream and deposits it deep in the abdominal area. According to a 2013 paper by researchers from the Methodist Hospital in Houston, the more belly fat you have, the more leptin you release. This stimulates the production of a group of proteins that usually only appears when you have a bacterial or viral infection. When your immune cells detect it, they crank up the inflammatory response.[20]

Gut microbes can also directly affect inflammation. In a European study published in *Diabetes,* researchers used antibiotic treatments to manipulate the gut microbiota in mice, slashing the numbers of harmful bacteria. By doing so, they created a more favorable balance of gut flora and were actually able to reduce metabolic endotoxemia, an inflammatory condition, in some of the mice. Those mice also gained less weight.[21]

> Diet is by far the biggest cause of chronic inflammation.

Diet, though, is by far the biggest cause of chronic inflammation. Saturated fats, found in red meat and dairy, have been found to promote inflammation in fatty tissue.[22] Consuming trans fats, a common ingredient in margarines, shortening, commercially baked goods, and fried fast food, also correlates with inflammation-influenced diseases. In an analysis of data from the long-running Nurses' Health Study, researchers at the Harvard School of Public Health found that women who consumed the most trans fatty acids had the highest markers of systemic cellular inflammation.[23]

One other type of fat, omega-6 fatty acids, is so closely associated with inflammation that it's used as a marker for inflammation in blood tests. One study, from the Center for Genetics, Nutrition and Health, in Washington, D.C., notes that our ancestors' diet contained an equal amount of omega-6 and omega-3 fatty acids, but now we eat almost 16 times more omega-6s than omega-3s. This same study demonstrated that lower ratios of omega-6s to omega-3s had beneficial effects for people with a number of different inflammatory diseases, from cardiovascular disease to rheumatoid arthritis to colorectal and breast cancers.[24]

On the flip side, foods that are high in fiber can cool inflammation, as can colorful fruits and vegetables rich in antioxidants and other vitamins and minerals. While the effects of dietary fats, fiber, and antioxidants on inflammation are well established, the roles of many other nutrients are still being studied. FODMAPs, for instance, might be implicated in chronic inflammation. Processed foods and refined carbohydrates have also been suspected of fanning the flames, but it's only now that a new theory explains the trait that might be responsible: carb density.

Triggers of Inflammation and Imbalance

Once hailed as marvels of modern engineering, processed foods and refined carbohydrates turn out to be ideal foods for "bad" bacteria. Two areas of very new research shed light on exactly what it is about these foods that cause us to gain both belly fat and belly issues—and exactly which carbs are the problem. Carb density, it appears, is a better predictor of whether or not a food is inflammatory than other ways of categorizing carbs. FODMAPs in foods are primary culprits in gas, bloating, and other GI symptoms.

Belly Alert! The Carb Density Discovery

Your digestive system breaks down carbohydrates into glucose, which is your cells' preferred fuel source. When this glucose enters your bloodstream, it's referred to as blood sugar or blood glucose. When blood sugar rises, beta cells in the pancreas release insulin, which escorts the blood sugar to cells to be burned for energy or stored for later. As your cells absorb and use it, the level of sugar in the blood drops. If blood sugar rises too fast, though, your cells can't absorb all of it and start to ignore insulin's instructions; this is called insulin resistance. In response, your pancreas pumps out more and more insulin to force cells to pay attention—until, exhausted by having to work overtime to produce extra insulin, the beta cells in your pancreas wear out entirely and insulin production stops altogether.

This is the pathway to type 2 diabetes. It's also the road to chronic inflammation and microbial imbalance. The extra high levels of insulin your pancreas produces make blood sugar levels fluctuate, triggering cravings for high-calorie foods, which lead you to pile on the pounds.

WHEN GUT FLORA GROWS WRONG

Maintaining a healthy gut microbiome may not just be a matter of which bacteria live in your gut or how many, but of where they live. Normally, fewer than 100,000 bacteria per milliliter reside in your small intestine, while more than 100 billion per milliliter congregate in your large intestine, where they help extract nutrition from hard-to-digest foods and protect our immune cells.

But in some people, the bacteria in their small intestine grow out of control, a condition known as small intestinal bacterial overgrowth (SIBO). SIBO causes gas, bloating, and diarrhea and has been associated with IBS, celiac disease, Crohn's disease, liver disease, and even fibromyalgia.[25] Remember, your small intestine is where most of the nutrients get extracted from food by your body. If extra bacteria live there, they may get to the nutrients before your cells do, which over time can lead to vitamin and mineral deficiencies. Plus, they expel excess gas, which is harder to move out of the small intestine than the large intestine, so you get bloated. They may also produce acid and other substances that irritate the small intestine, causing diarrhea and other problems. Bacteria in the small intestine also get to the bile before bile is able to do its job of helping your body digest fats. So SIBO can contribute to faulty fat digestion too.

Antibiotics can control the symptoms for a short while. Starving these bacteria by removing their favorite food sources, FODMAPs, as you'll do on the 21-Day Tummy diet, may solve the problem more permanently.

Since it's the cumulative effect of the carbohydrates that leads to chronic inflammation and an imbalance in your gut flora, new science suggests that what's most important is how much carbohydrate is in a food per weight. This is the food's carb density.

Carbohydrates are counted in grams, and carb density is determined by weighing the amount of carb grams in a food compared to its other ingredients. For instance, let's consider the potato. The potato is a heavy food; just one small potato weighs in at 170 grams. Most of those 170 grams, though, are water weight. Only about 23 percent consists of non-fibrous carbs. Thus, the potato is not actually carb-dense. In fact, Kate and I call potatoes (and other foods with a carb density less than 30 percent) carb-light, and we've included them on the 21-Day Tummy meal plan. A plain rice cake, by contrast, only weighs 9 grams. But almost 80 percent of it is carbohydrate—now that's carb dense! Plus, because rice cakes don't fill you up, it's easy to eat more than one at each sitting, which exacerbates the issue.

Ian Spreadbury, a researcher at Queen's University in Ontario, Canada, proposed the carb density hypothesis in 2012. He noted that "modern foods" containing flour and sugar are carb-dense, while "ancestral foods" that our hunter-gatherer forebears would have eaten are not. Carb sources on hunter-gatherer diets include root tubers (like potatoes, cassava, jicamas, and yams), leafy vegetables (like lettuce, spinach, and kale), and fruit (like kiwis, oranges, and bananas). These plants store their carbohydrates in cells that have walls made of fiber, which are thought to remain intact during cooking. As a result, their carbs are "locked in" while they pass through the esophagus and stomach, only being released into the bloodstream after stomach acids and other digestive juices start to break down the cell walls.

By contrast, the carbs in flour- and sugar-based foods are available to the bacteria in your mouth right away (contributing to cavities), and therefore represent a much higher carb concentration than the upper GI tract is designed for. This may lead to an overgrowth of bacteria in the small intestine, which can cause malnutrition and digestive symptoms. It may also, Spreadbury believes, cause the microbiota in the stomach and small intestine to become inflamed. And once your microbiome becomes inflamed, it releases toxins that can create systemic inflammation.[27] As you know by now, that not only leads to a tubby tummy but to a wide range of health problems, including type 2 diabetes, heart disease, cancer, and of course, belly-roiling digestive issues.

The carb density hypothesis helps to explain why the simple carbs in fruit don't cause the same type of swings in blood sugar you get from table sugar, and why some starchy foods, like potatoes and bananas, don't seem to contribute to inflammation, even though they cause blood sugar to spike.

It also explains the success of so-called Paleo or primal diets, modern re-creations of the hunter-gatherer diet that advocate the removal of all refined foods, including grains. Not many clinical studies have been done on Paleo diets, and those that have are pretty small—but their results are suggestive. In all of them, subjects who followed Paleo diets lost weight, shrank their bellies, and/or significantly improved blood sugar, blood pressure, and other cardiovascular risk factors.[28, 29] And they did better on all these measures than people who followed a Mediterranean-style diet, currently considered the gold standard of heart-healthy, diabetes-friendly, antiaging diets.[30, 31] The Paleo diets even proved to be more satisfying. In the most recent study, subjects were randomly divided into two groups—one followed a Paleo diet, one a Mediterranean-like diet—and were asked to record their satiety levels throughout the day. While the Paleo group actually consumed fewer calories, they reported feeling just as full as the Mediterranean group.[32]

The 21-Day Tummy eating plan takes the best aspect of the Paleo diets—the avoidance of carb-dense foods—and

> "Modern foods" containing flour and sugar are carb-dense, while "ancestral foods" are not.

(continued on page 42)

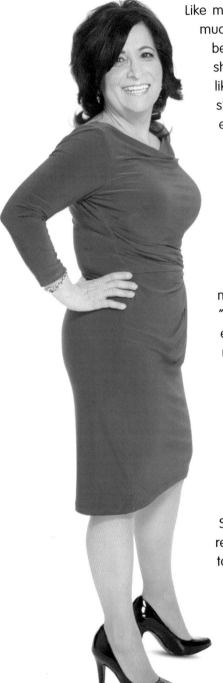

Like many women, Dorothy Nuzzo didn't like her belly very much. "It was big and in my way all the time," she complained before she started the 21-Day Tummy meal plan. When she sat, she felt the weight of her stomach pressing up, likely a cause of her frequent gas and heartburn. When she lay down to sleep, she found it tough to roll over. And every pound showed on her petite frame.

After 21-Day Tummy? Heartburn and gas are no longer a part of Dorothy's life; they are 100 percent gone. Her body aches have decreased, she's more flexible, and she was able to go from 3.8 miles per hour on the treadmill to 4.5 miles. "I feel much lighter," she says. "I can move much easier, and I feel much more comfortable in my clothes. I feel that my belly is a lot flatter."

Lightening—and Lighting—Up at Midlife

In addition, she exclaims, "I lost more than 6 pounds, and for someone my size—I'm only 4'10"—that's a lot of weight. It shows right away."

The best part? "I was always full. I never felt hungry, and I felt good about eating healthy foods."

Going out to dinner is Dorothy's favorite way to relax. She says it wasn't a problem to stick with the diet in restaurants. "I never cheated. If I saw cake, I didn't want to eat it because I was full. That was the biggest surprise. I was thrilled by that, actually."

Unlike other diets, on which she lost weight but didn't feel good, the 21-Day Tummy plan caused her energy levels to soar, her overall well-being to improve, and her self-confidence to fly off the charts. "All in all, I am feeling great!" she proclaims.

The happiest news? Dorothy has learned exactly

what foods she should avoid to stay this way. Onions, bread, and soft cheeses like ricotta are among Dorothy's personal Belly Bullies. "The heartburn and bloating come back big time when I eat them. The diet changed my eating habits and made me much more aware of what I am consuming. I can evaluate if what I am about to eat is worth the calories and/or discomfort."

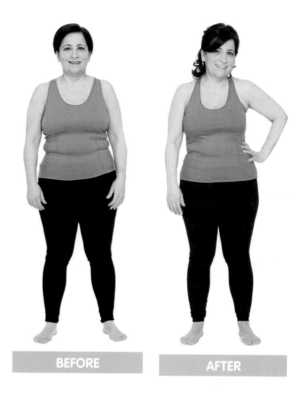

BEFORE　　AFTER

Dorothy Nuzzo

Age 55

Lost 6½ POUNDS and 2¼ BELLY INCHES in 21 days!

Proudest accomplishments: Wasn't tempted by cake; walked farther and faster

Favorite meal: Belly Soother Smoothie

(continued from page 39)

improves upon it. Whereas the Paleo diets are accidentally carb-light, Kate specifically designed the 21-Day Tummy menus to take advantage of this revolutionary discovery.

While most grains are, in fact, carb-dense, a handful have a much lighter carb load and play an important role in the 21-Day Tummy diet. Since researchers at MIT have demonstrated that carbs act as natural antidepressants by boosting levels of the feel-good brain chemical serotonin, we want to fill up on healthy carbs in proper portions.[33] By focusing on carb-light grains, the 21-Day Tummy meal plan gives you the benefits of carb-cutting without the moodiness.

> Eat too many of these rapidly fermentable carbs, and your bacteria work overtime producing gas.

Plus, the 21-Day Tummy diet adds other foods that help fight inflammation, such as magnesium-rich fruits and vegetables. Kate also took into account the fact that some vegetables, fruits, and nuts can make our bellies bloat. I want your stomach to feel as good as it's going to look, which is why the 21-Day Tummy diet restricts another category of carbohydrates: FODMAPs. I quickly discovered that I was particularly sensitive to certain FODMAPs and needed the soothing aspects of carb-light and magnesium-rich foods. Once I started eating the 21-Day Tummy way, my belly bloat (and extra belly fat) disappeared.

Belly Alert! Rapidly Fermentable Carbs, or FODMAPs

When your midafternoon slump hits (which, for some of us early risers, usually happens midmorning!), is your first inclination to reach for a cookie? Since carbs are digested most rapidly, and sugars are the fastest type of carb to digest, that cookie can indeed give you a quick burst of energy. But not only is the cookie carb-dense, it contains some types of sugars (or saccharides) that your body can't digest very well. So these sugars often move along your digestive tract to the large intestine, where they become food for your gut bacteria, leading to gas.

Bacteria "digest" food by fermentation. Chemically speaking, fermentation occurs when a sugar is broken down into an acid. Lactose, for instance, is first broken down into the simpler sugars glucose and galactose. The glucose, in turn, is broken down into lactic acid, which consists of hydrogen and oxygen; the carbon combines with some of the oxygen to become carbon dioxide, a gas.

You see how an excess of fermentation can lead to excess acid and gas in your GI system. And, just as you digest some foods more rapidly than others, your bacteria ferment some sugars more rapidly than others. Eat too many of these rapidly fermentable carbs, and your bacteria work overtime producing gas. These carbs also draw water into the intestine, which can cause diarrhea or constipation or both (a hallmark of IBS).

TUMMY **TWISTER** OR **TAMER?**
Fermented Foods

There's a difference between fermentable foods and fermented foods. Some fermented foods are good for your tummy; others can create problems for certain people. Many different types of bacteria can start the fermentation process; so can many different kinds of yeasts, molds, and fungi. And not all of them live in our gut. When these bacteria or yeast are combined with different foods, the results can be delicious—think wine, cheese, vinegar, miso, yogurt, kefir, sauerkraut, kimchi, and pickles. (Pickling is, in fact, a form of fermentation.)

To make yogurt, for instance, you combine milk with *Lactobacillus bulgaricus* and *Streptococcus thermophiles*. These bacteria break down some of the lactose in the milk, so what remains may be easier for your stomach to process. Thus, fermented foods are often considered "probiotic foods" that are good for your gut.

Be careful, though! Many fermented foods also contain FODMAPs, which may negate their digestive benefits. Kimchi, for instance—a spicy Korean dish that can be served with just about anything from noodles to stir-fries—is usually made with cabbage and scallions. Napa cabbage is high in FODMAPs, as is the white part of the scallion; if you stick with kimchi made with common cabbage and the green part of the scallion, though, you'll be A-OK. Similarly, if you like kefir, a fermented drink of milk and kefir grains, check the label to make sure it's low in lactose (most are).

If you have a sweet tooth like me, fermented foods can take a little getting used to; the acids produced by the fermentation give them a sour taste. But I learned to love my Greek yogurt plain (well, at least I learned to combine it with belly-friendly sweeteners)—and I love even more how good it makes my belly feel.

FODMAPs may also contribute to inflammation. According to a 2010 study in the journal *Toxicology*, when certain gut bacteria ferment some FODMAPs, they produce toxic metabolites in addition to acid and gas.[34] These metabolites may disrupt signaling mechanisms in cells around the body, triggering an inflammatory response and changing the balance of microflora in the gut. This, as we've seen, can cause belly fat as well as belly bloating; it's what happened to me!

There are several different types of rapidly fermentable carbs, as indicated by the acronym by which they are known— **FODMAPs.** This stands for:

Fermentable
Oligosaccharides: fructans and galacto-oligosaccharides (GOS)
Disaccharides: lactose
Monosaccharides: fructose
And
Polyols: sugar alcohols such as sorbitol, mannitol, maltitol, and xylitol

You may already know or suspect you're sensitive to certain foods. As excited as I was to start the 21-Day Tummy diet, I was afraid that I'd find I was lactose intolerant. A glass of milk with dinner has been part of my life since I can remember. (A life without cheese is as horrifying a thought as a life without chocolate.) I worried these favorites were my problem.

FODMAPs lurk in a wide variety of foods, even healthy ones like pears and cauliflower. But don't worry! Just because a food is on our Belly Bully list doesn't mean you can never eat it again. It's not the food your gut reacts badly to; it's the FODMAPs in them. And there are a few things to keep in mind about FODMAPs:

1. **People react differently to different FODMAPs.** Almost everyone has a problem with GOS, because the human body lacks the enzyme to break

apart the chains of galactose fibers that make up this FODMAP. That's why beans and legumes, the primary food source of GOS, are so widely known as gas-producers. Fructose doesn't affect everyone the same way, though, so whereas you might be fine gorging on foods high in fructose, such as honey, I get a stomachache since my tummy is sensitive to it.

2. **FODMAPs have a cumulative effect on your GI tract.** Your digestive system can handle a lot. Even people who are lactose-intolerant are usually fine with a splash or two of milk in their coffee. But the more FODMAPs you feed your bacteria, the more gas they produce and the more problems you have. Remember—FODMAPs are carbs, so carb density matters here, too. The more carb-dense a FODMAP-containing food is (whole wheat cereal, for instance, is 70 percent carbs, while white bread is 50 percent), the more likely it may be to cause digestive symptoms. And foods that contain more than one FODMAP (such as apples or snow peas) have the potential to be the biggest troublemakers on the digestive tract.

> FODMAPs lurk in a wide variety of foods, even healthy ones like pears and cauliflower.

3. **FODMAP-containing foods are not inherently unhealthy or fattening.** Far from it! In fact, many of them are nutrient-packed and fiber-rich, so you don't want to cut them out of your diet forever, unless they are a real issue for you. We've taken them all out of the 21-Day Tummy diet because we want to give your gut a break. But after that, we'll lead you through the steps to identify what your specific Belly Bullies are so you know just which foods you can tolerate and in what amounts. (In my case, that means bring on the milk!)

The concept of FODMAPs is new. Even many dietitians and gastroenterologists are unclear about the nuances of creating a low-FODMAP diet. A lot of research still needs to be done to chart what foods contain which FODMAPs and in what quantities, and how they interact with other factors to affect digestive diseases. One group that has been on the forefront of this research is the Department of Gastroenterology at Australia's Monash University.

Peter R. Gibson, MD, the head of this department, has led the effort to measure FODMAPs in food as a way of determining an effective treatment plan for IBS. In a review of common approaches to managing IBS symptoms, he found that "the greatest body of evidence is for the low-FODMAP diet, which improves symptoms in at least 74 percent of patients with IBS."[36] And it's not just IBS sufferers who find relief on a low-FODMAP diet. People with celiac disease and IBD who experience gas and bloating, abdominal pain, constipation, and diarrhea benefit from cutting out FODMAPs.[37]

***

Now that you've learned how hard your body—and your belly—works to keep you fueled up and ready to go, I

GLUTEN AND YOUR 21-DAY TUMMY

A protein composite most common in foods made of wheat and some other grains, gluten makes dough doughy. For people with celiac disease, gluten is downright toxic. When they eat it, their immune systems release antibodies that attack the lining of the small intestine, preventing the absorption of nutrients. Symptoms range considerably and contain any combination of bloating, diarrhea, abdominal pain, irritability, anemia, joint pain, skin rash, and muscle cramps.

Other people are gluten intolerant or gluten sensitive. They may be able to handle small amounts of gluten, but if they have too much, woe is their tummy. A 2011 study demonstrated that gluten triggers an inflammatory response in these folks, but they do not suffer long-term damage to their intestines.[35] The most common symptoms include excess gas, constipation, and diarrhea, but some people have also reported fatigue, headaches, depression, and brain fog.

It's become trendy these days to go gluten-free, and many people who have report that their digestive systems clear up, their weight drops, and their energy levels soar. This might be a sign that their symptoms were caused by gluten—or, it might just be because they're no longer eating carb-heavy foods. Because many of these foods also happen to be carb-dense, the 21-Day Tummy plan already cuts them out. Our menus can easily be made completely gluten-free (we've made notes in the meal plan accordingly), so they're suitable whether you have celiac disease or gluten intolerance.

want you to take a moment to say thank you. Too often, we think of our bodies as the enemy, especially that hated beer gut or tummy pooch. But all too often, that attitude leads us down a path to deprivation diets, punishing workouts, pill popping, and other "shortcuts" to weight loss that might work for a little while. These approaches take a toll on your body; some can even be dangerous to your health; and a lot of them backfire, causing you to regain all the weight you lost and then some. Plus, they're just no fun!

With the 21-Day Tummy plan, we're going to give our bodies, and ourselves, a break. Remember that your goal is to soothe and shrink your belly, so that you never again need to experience the five digestive disasters we're going to learn about next.

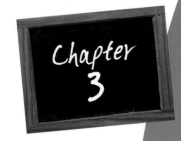

Dieting Away
Digestive
Disasters

Raging heartburn, embarrassing gas, running to the restroom at work and hoping for some, well, alone time—none of that is fun. So why do millions of us put up with it?

You may think it's normal. Or you may feel like it's worth a little pain to be able to eat whatever you want. I have one friend who takes a sort of perverse pride in his "cast-iron stomach." He boasts that he can handle the gas pain and cramps he gets from eating the spiciest street food in Thailand, all-you-can-eat kebabs in Dubai, and "real" enchiladas smothered in rich mole sauce in Mexico. "I'm not going to let my stomach problems stop me from eating what I want," he says defiantly.

While I admire his adventurous spirit and understand his determination not let digestive issues control his life, wouldn't it be far more empowering to prevent them in the first place? I promise, preventing tummy troubles doesn't mean never eating for pleasure again. Instead, a little understanding can go a long way. So let's take a closer look at the five common digestive disasters that the 21-Day Tummy diet soothes.

Enemies One Through Five

The following GI issues plague people from Maine to Oregon, from Toronto to Vancouver, from the United States and Canada to industrialized countries around the world. They are the most common chronic tummy troubles—and while they are easy to diagnose, their causes are sometimes tough to tease out because there are so many possible factors that can contribute.

The 21-Day Tummy diet is designed to solve these five stomach problems:

1. Gas and bloating

2. Heartburn and acid reflux

3. Constipation

4. Diarrhea

5. Irritable bowel syndrome (IBS)

These conditions are not only embarrassing, but they may signal more serious problems. Even worse, some of these conditions can turn into serious, even life-threatening, diseases if you don't treat them promptly.

To make matters even more confusing, these five issues often appear together. Do you alternate between the rock-hard feces of constipation and the rushing watery excrement of diarrhea? You may have IBS, a constellation of digestive problems. Look back at your answers to the Digestion Quiz in Chapter 1 and think about how many of these five you experience, how often, and to what extent. Share this information with your doctor, or a gastroenterologist, especially if you suspect you have IBS.

The good news, though, is that you don't need to choose whether you'd rather suffer from heartburn or gas. All of these conditions may be signs of inflammation and microbial imbalance, and are inextricably linked to excess weight and poor diets. So if you follow the nourishing 21-Day Tummy plan to cool inflammation and balance your gut bacteria, you can blast all of these symptoms and your belly fat at the same time.

Disaster #1: Gas and Bloating

Here's a statistic you won't want to share at the next cocktail party: The average person releases gas (through burping or farting) from 10 to 20 times per day, according to the American College of Gastroenterology.[1] Since we often pass gas silently when we're eating, sleeping, or sitting on the toilet, we usually don't even notice. But excess gas is hard to ignore. When that gas builds up in your stomach or small intestine, you feel it as bloating or as pain in your abdomen.

Estimates suggest that between 16 and 30 percent of the American population experience frequent bloating (at least 3 days a month for at least 3 months), according to a 2011 study published in the journal *Gastroenterology & Hepatology*.[2] The same study found that 90 percent of people with irritable bowel syndrome (especially those who have more constipation than diarrhea) endured bloating. Similar studies conducted outside the United States indicate that rates are comparable worldwide and

IF YOU HAVE OTHER GI ISSUES

An entire field of medicine is devoted to gastrointestinal diseases that extend beyond our top five digestive disorders. When I asked Kate to create the 21-Day Tummy diet, we chose to focus on these five common conditions because their causes are similar enough that one diet could treat or prevent them all.

If you have other, more serious GI issues, like inflammatory bowel disease (such as ulcerative colitis or Crohn's disease), gallstones, or peptic ulcers, you need an individualized treatment plan managed by your physician or other health care provider. But by all means, give them a copy of this book! The 21-Day Tummy way of eating may be able to help relieve some of your symptoms, and your health care provider can tell you if you need to make any modifications.

If you have celiac disease or gluten intolerance, you'll see that the 21-Day Tummy eating plan is largely gluten free; we've pointed out the few spots where gluten might sneak in if you're not careful. If you are lactose intolerant, don't be scared off by the dairy products you see in the meal plan. Give the 21-Day Tummy diet a try—you may be surprised to find that you don't have to avoid all dairy in order to prevent your symptoms.

that women are more than twice as likely to suffer from bloating than men.[3]

What Causes Gas and Bloating?

What's in digestive gas? It's mostly nitrogen, hydrogen, and carbon dioxide, with some oxygen and sometimes methane. Some of these substances are also found in the air we breathe. That's right. Gas is basically air that happens to be trapped in our digestive tract. When we eat and drink, we naturally swallow some air, but some behaviors cause us to swallow more than usual:

1. Wolfing down food
2. Using a straw
3. Chewing gum
4. Sucking on hard candy
5. Drinking carbonated beverages (including draft beer)

The sugar or sweeteners in gum, candy, and most carbonated beverages can be problematic, so you won't find them on the 21-Day Tummy plan. And taking at least 20 minutes to eat each meal can also encourage you to chew more and enjoy your food, for which your digestive system will thank you.

Adding to the outside air we've trapped in our GI tract is the gas given off by our gut flora. When undigestible carbohydrates reach the large intestine, some bacteria start to break them down, producing hydrogen and carbon dioxide in the process. Other microbes in the large intestine use this hydrogen to produce methane gas or hydrogen sulfide, which is released as flatulence.[4]

Sometimes, flatulence is innocuous. If it's quiet and doesn't smell, it pretty much goes unnoticed. But what's with the smelly kind? That foul smell is caused by the presence of sulfur gases.[5] We get these sulfur gases if the undigested food in the large intestine starts to decompose. Food decomposing. Doesn't that sound awful? I don't want my food doing anything that a dead squirrel does in a forest.

The irony here is that often healthy fiber-filled foods are what's decomposing. Remember, the foods that cause

you to bloat may differ from the ones that give me grief. That's because you and I have different types of bacteria in our guts. But some types of carbs—those pesky FODMAPs—have been identified as most likely to cause excess gas for many people, so Kate and I deemed the foods that contain them Belly Bullies even though they are healthy. Foods that often cause gas include beans, onions, garlic, cauliflower, apples, pears, apricots, nectarines, blackberries, and lactose in dairy products.

In some people, laxatives (which may contain fibrous bulking agents) and antibiotics (which disrupt healthy gut bacteria) can also lead to excess gas. Some diseases, such as ovarian cancer, cause gas and bloating. (That's why it's important to tell your doctor about your digestive symptoms, even if you're embarrassed.)

Bloating, that uncomfortable feeling of fullness in the abdomen, is usually caused by too much gas buildup in the stomach or small intestine. But it's not just gas that contributes to bloating. Eating a lot of fatty foods can also do it, since fats tend to be the slowest types of foods to empty out of your belly. Intestinal obstructions—usually caused by diseases such as colon cancer or as a side effect of having had multiple operations, internal hernias, or bands of internal scar tissue—can also make it harder for food to leave your stomach, producing bloat.

If you feel like you have water weight in your lower belly,

you're probably right. FODMAPs and salty foods draw water into the colon, while sluggish bowels trap water. Changes in hormone levels before and during menstruation can also lead some women to retain water, which also feels like bloat.

How Can You Prevent or Treat Gas and Bloating?

Once gas has accumulated in your digestive tract, there's not much you can do other than pass it out of your system. Most of the gas in your esophagus and stomach is passed by burping, the gas from your large intestine by farting. Some gas is partially absorbed in your small intestine; some remains trapped in your stomach and intestines, causing bloating.

Exercise helps force out trapped gas by promoting movement in the muscles of the GI tract. While any kind of physical activity can help, the combination of aerobic exercise and core strengthening moves in the 21-Day Tummy workout specifically target the muscles that can move food and gas along more efficiently.

You can also try over-the-counter supplements, although they have not yet been scientifically proven to be effective in treating gas and bloating. Some, like lactase supplements, provide the body with enzymes needed to digest specific FOD-MAPs, so that they don't pass through to the colon to feed the bacteria there. Simethicone (like Gas-X) is an antifoaming agent that helps break the gas into smaller gas bubbles so they move more easily out of your digestive tract, while activated charcoal, sold as tablets, has a huge surface area to help absorb excess intestinal gas.

Otherwise, the best way to treat gas is to prevent it. In

LAUGHING GAS

- What's a small part of an English teacher's colon? The semicolon.
- What do you get if you eat beans and onions? Teargas.
- What do you call someone who doesn't fart in public? A private tutor.
- Did you hear about the constipated accountant? He couldn't budget.
- Incontinence Hotline. Can you hold, please?

addition to avoiding the foods and behaviors listed on pages 52 and 53, it can also help to eat smaller, more frequent meals, which are easier for your body to break down efficiently. And, when you smoke, you inhale some excess air, so quitting smoking can reduce gas, not to mention help you avoid heart disease and cancer.

> Once gas has accumulated in your digestive tract, there's not much you can do other than pass it.

But, of course, the key to preventing excess gas and bloating is the 21-Day Tummy diet. On this plan, we've taken out all the FODMAPs and fatty foods that could possibly bother your belly, and replaced them with delicious low-FODMAP fruits, vegetables, and grains and satisfying healthy fats.

Disaster #2: Heartburn and Acid Reflux

Ever experience a burning sensation in your throat or pressure in your chest after a big lunch or dinner? Is the pain worse at night or when you lie down? That feeling is what's commonly referred to as heartburn or acid indigestion. Heartburn is caused by acid reflux, which is the regurgitation of liquid or food.

Many people experience slight heartburn a couple times a year; that's nothing to worry about. It's frequent heartburn that's concerning. The National Institutes of Health and the Canadian Digestive Health Foundation report that a whopping 60 million Americans and 5 million Canadians experience reflux symptoms at least once a week.[6,7] If you experience heartburn more than twice a week, you should see your doctor, because frequent heartburn can lead to gastroesophageal reflux disease, more commonly known as GERD.

GERD, a chronic digestive disorder, involves frequent acid reflux. In addition to heartburn, reflux may cause a dry cough, hoarseness or sore throat, agitated vocal cords, chest pain, and difficulty swallowing. GERD is one of the most common digestive disorders, accounting for 17.5 percent of all digestive system diagnoses in the outpatient setting.[8] A 2010 study published in the medical journal *Digestive Diseases and Sciences* found that the rate of GERD-related doctor visits nearly doubled from 1995 to 2006. The article suggests that this influx of visits may be related to an increase in excess weight in recent years.[9] I believe it! The standard American diet that's responsible for our increasingly overweight population also leads to the imbalance of gut flora and chronic inflammation that can cause acid reflux and GERD.

KNOWLEDGE NIBBLES

Even if you never experience heartburn, you might still have GERD. In some people, acid reflux affects the throat or lungs more than the chest, so your symptoms resemble those of a cold (sore throat and cough).

GERD, in turn, can lead to Barrett's esophagus, a serious condition that occurs when the cells of the esophagus become damaged. Over time these cellular changes can lead to esophageal cancer, the sixth most common cause of cancer-related deaths worldwide.

What Causes Heartburn and Acid Reflux?

Your lower esophageal sphincter (LES), a circular band of muscle around the bottom part of the esophagus, relaxes when you swallow. This allows food and liquid to flow down into your stomach, after which your esophageal sphincter closes again. If your esophageal sphincter relaxes too much, though, partially digested food and liquid, along with stomach acid, can flow back up into your esophagus. That, as Kate explained to me, is acid reflux, and it's every bit as unpleasant as it sounds.

Anything that increases pressure on your abdomen can push your stomach contents up into the esophagus, which is why eating too much is a prime cause of heartburn. Having a big belly, whether from obesity or pregnancy, also does it.

Your chances of acid reflux also increase if something damages your LES. When you smoke, chemicals in the tobacco weaken the LES. With a hiatal hernia, the upper part of the stomach pushes through an opening in the diaphragm and into the chest; that opening, or hiatus, normally serves as a backup sphincter to the LES, so when it is blocked, the LES is more easily overwhelmed.

Many commonly prescribed medications can also impair the LES or increase acid production in the stomach (both of which can lead to more heartburn), including:

- antibiotics, such as tetracycline

- aspirin

- beta-blockers for high blood pressure or heart disease, such as Inderal (propranolol)

- bisphosphonates for osteoporosis, such as Fosamax (alendronate), Boniva (ibandronate), and Actonel (risedronate)

- calcium channel blockers for high blood pressure, such as Procardia (nifedipine)

- certain bronchodilators for asthma, such as albuterol

- hormone replacement therapy (HRT), with a combination of estrogen and progesterone

- nonsteroidal anti-inflammatory drugs (NSAIDs) such as ibuprofen and naproxen

- sedatives for anxiety, such as Valium (diazepam) or Ativan (lorezepam)

IS IT HEARTBURN, A HEART ATTACK, OR PEPTIC ULCERS?

Because the nerves in your chest don't clearly signal to your brain where pain might come from, heartburn is frequently confused with other types of discomfort—especially that caused by heart attacks and by peptic ulcers.

The chest pain caused by heartburn can feel very similar to a heart attack. But heart-related pain usually only lasts about 10 minutes while heartburn can go on for hours. Also, heartburn symptoms usually get worse when you lie down or bend over, while pain from a heart attack is exacerbated by exercise or stress.

Like acid reflux, peptic ulcers also cause a burning sensation. But that burning sensation occurs in the stomach, rather than the chest, and usually on an empty stomach. And whereas heartburn symptoms can often be relieved by changing positions (such as standing up), ulcer pain remains.

If you experience chest tightness or feel very weak or faint, please go to the emergency room right away to get checked out. If your symptoms are mild or pass when you rest, you can skip the ER but I suggest that you see your doctor as soon as you can.

(continued on page 59)

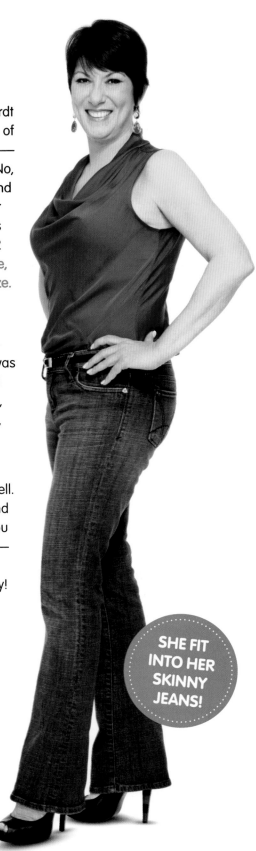

Phyllis Gebhardt

Prior to the 21-Day Tummy diet, Phyllis Gebhardt regularly experienced a not-so-fun combination of nausea, heartburn, bloating, and abdominal pain— all that on top of a "family birthright of constipation." No, thank you! She wanted to reduce her symptoms and her waistline, and she did just that, getting off all her medications. In just 3 weeks, Phyllis lost 2½ pounds and 6 inches from all over her body, including 2 inches from her belly. In the weeks and months since, she's continued to lose weight, dropping a whole size.

Q: What motivated you to try the diet?

A: Before the plan, I was having really terrible heartburn in the morning, and my digestive system just was not predictable at all. I have not had heartburn at all since I started this diet. All systems are working well, and I like my belly a whole lot more. It's a little flatter, and it doesn't hurt.

Q: What did you learn from the diet?

A: I had gotten really, really, far away from eating well. I had forgotten how easy it is to incorporate fruits and vegetables in your life and how good they taste if you have the right recipes. You don't even need to cook— my favorite discovery was frozen grapes. Just as good as ice cream, and they don't bother my tummy!

Q: What did you like most about the diet?

A: It was easy to find everything that I needed and easy to make everything. I don't really feel like it's a diet, it's just a way of eating that I plan to maintain. And I fit into my small jeans without wiggling!

SHE FIT INTO HER SKINNY JEANS!

(continued from page 57)

Finally, while the research is mixed, many people do find that certain foods trigger heartburn. Common culprits include coffee, chocolate, soda, alcohol, meat, dairy, spicy foods, fried foods, and acidic foods.

How Can You Treat or Prevent Heartburn and Acid Reflux?

You probably already carry with you the simplest treatment for heartburn: chewing gum. While it cannot prevent the stomach acid from entering your esophagus, chewing gum stimulates the production of saliva, which is alkaline. Thus, it neutralizes the acids that cause the sensation of burning. (Remember, though, that chewing gum can cause excess gas.) Another simple way to dampen the acidity? Drink a glass of water. In a Greek study, water worked faster than several ulcer medications to raise the pH level in your gut and relieve heartburn symptoms.[10]

Changes in your body position can also help relieve heartburn symptoms. Standing up straight (instead of slouching) after meals can help food and acid stay in your stomach instead of traveling up into your esophagus. Sleeping on your side instead of your stomach, and elevating your head and upper body when you lie down, are both time-honored remedies for heartburn.

If these no-cost solutions don't work, there are always antacids. These medications, including Alka-Seltzer, Pepto-Bismol, and milk of magnesia, all work well to neutralize stomach acid but can cause constipation, diarrhea, or other side effects. Histamine antagonists like Pepcid, Tagamet, and

TUMMY TWISTER OR TAMER? Acidic Food

In almost every list of "the worst foods for digestion," you'll find acidic foods like oranges and tomatoes. These are commonly thought to cause heartburn, which occurs when stomach acid rises up through the lower esophageal sphincter (LES), the doorway between your stomach and your esophagus. Protein-rich meals increase the LES pressure (a good thing) while fatty meals tend to lower the LES pressure and therefore contribute to acid reflux (a bad thing). Studies have shown, though, that acidic foods don't have any effect on LES pressure and don't cause heartburn symptoms . . . which is why you'll see that oranges and tomatoes are allowed on the 21-Day Tummy diet.[11]

That being said, if you have severe acid reflux that hasn't been treated and has irritated the esophagus, acidic foods can be like "salt in the wound." Ouch! So if you find that oranges or tomatoes do make your heartburn feel worse, replace them with other fruits.

Zantac and proton pump inhibitors like Prevacid, Prilosec, and Zegerid work to reduce the production of acid in the stomach. These also often cause side effects, including chest tightness, fever, and fatigue. Proton pump inhibitors can also contribute to small intestinal bacterial overgrowth.[12]

To prevent heartburn, your doctor may tell you to stop smoking, lose weight, eat smaller and more frequent meals, and avoid lying down for at least 3 hours following a meal. And, of course, try to avoid the foods listed on page 59 that may trigger heartburn. Many of these foods, you'll see, also happen to be Belly Bullies, so if you follow the 21-Day Tummy diet, you won't have any trouble with them.

Disaster #3: Constipation

While regularity varies from person to person, doctors consider you constipated if you haven't had a bowel movement for more than 3 days or if you experience difficulty or pain when passing a hardened stool. Constipation means passing stool that is smaller than usual, straining to have a bowel movement, having a feeling that there's waste that didn't come out, or needing enemas, suppositories, or laxatives in order to be regular.

Like most digestive issues, occasional constipation is no big deal. Chronic constipation, however, can be a symptom of something more serious. If your constipation lasts more than

3 weeks or if you have abdominal pain, bloody or thin stools, rectal pain, unexpected weight loss, or constipation that alternates with diarrhea, call your doctor. These may be signs of irritable bowel syndrome (IBS), colon cancer, or anal fissures.

Chronic constipation can lead to complications. When you strain to go to the bathroom, the pressure may result in painful hemorrhoids. And a 2012 study from the American College of Gastroenterology found that people who suffer from chronic constipation may be at a greater risk for colon cancer.[14]

Clearly, constipation is not innocuous. And with 63 million North Americans affected at last count,[15] I'm hardly alone in looking for a way to end this problem for good.

> Anything that slows the passage of food through the GI tract can cause constipation.

What Causes Constipation?

The longer it takes food to move through the digestive tract, the more water the large intestine removes, making stool that is hard and dry and tough to pass. How long it takes your digestive tract to digest food varies, depending on what and how much you've eaten and the bacteria in your gut.

Anything that slows the passage of food through the GI tract can cause constipation. Stress causes our GI muscles to clench up, making it harder for food to move through. When we exercise, our breathing and heart rate pick up, stimulating our intestinal muscles to contract and move food along; sitting like a slug, on the other hand, makes our digestive system sluggish.

Our standard American diet is to blame here, too, of course. Fried foods and unhealthy fats can be difficult to digest. But the biggest problem is what we're not eating: fiber.

But wait. If foods that are difficult to digest cause constipation, how can something your body can't digest at all help? Undigested fiber, which acts like a cleaning sponge for the digestive system, is the exception to the rule. Like a pipe cleaner, fiber scrubs out food and waste particles and soaks

SEEKING REGULARITY: FIBER SUPPLEMENTS

Most of us are only getting about 15 grams of fiber a day, a far cry from the recommended 25 to 38 grams. It's tempting to reach for a pill to make up the difference, but beware: Not all fiber supplements are created equal. Psyllium seed husk and wheat bran increase stool weight the most, giving it just the heft it needs for your digestive muscles to grab on and move it along.[16, 17]

Inulin, by contrast, has zero effect on stool weight, according to researchers at the University of Minnesota.[18] Also called chicory root extract, inulin is used as a fiber supplement and frequently added to cereals, breads, and other food products to increase the fiber content. "It's completely fermented," noted study author Joanne Slavin, "so by the end of the ride, there's nothing left." Guess what? That rapid fermentation means it's a FODMAP, a prime source of fuel for the bacteria in your gut. While some of the bacteria inulin feeds may be good for gut health (which is why inulin is considered a prebiotic), even friendly bacteria can give off gas. Whether inulin is a problem for you depends on how much you eat and which bacteria you have in your gut.

With the 21-Day Tummy eating plan, you won't need fiber supplements. Kate worked hard to ensure that you get your 25 grams of fiber from delicious, real, low-FODMAP foods like chia seeds.

up water. Fiber adds bulk to your stool, giving the muscles of your GI tract something to grab on to, so they can keep moving food along.

The other culprit? Lack of water. When you're constipated, your stool is hard and dry. You want to drink enough to keep your stool softer and easier to pass.

Medications with sedative or diuretic effects can cause constipation; these include narcotics, antidepressants, and calcium channel blockers. Medical conditions that generally slow down the body's processes, such as hypothyroidism and depression, or that cause neurological damage, such as Parkinson's disease, multiple sclerosis, and diabetes, can also contribute. Hormonal changes in pregnancy also slow down your digestive system, as do disruptions to your circadian rhythm when you travel. And when you have hemorrhoids or anal fissures, which may be caused by constipation, the pain may cause you to resist the urge to go to the bathroom, which can cause more constipation.

How Can You Treat or Prevent Constipation?

To start, let me warn you against reaching for laxatives. If you take them frequently, over time, your intestinal muscles become weaker, which causes constipation. Stool softeners, which act on the stool itself, are safer but should not be used on a regular basis. If you find yourself using a laxative more than a few times a year, and diet changes aren't helping, visit a doctor to find a more sustainable treatment.

Non-pharmacological treatments for constipation include drinking more water, increasing physical activity, and reducing stress. And if you feel the urge to go, then go! When you resist, you disrupt the normal nerve reflex that helps you pass stool easily and stool backs up in your large intestine.

Perhaps the most important thing you can do to prevent and treat constipation, though, is to make sure you get enough fiber in your diet. The *Dietary Guidelines for Americans*—a set of recommendations for a healthful diet issued jointly by the U.S. Department of Agriculture and Department of Health and Human Services and generally also followed by Canadians—calls for 25 grams of fiber per day for women and 38 grams for men.[19] Foods such as fresh fruits and vegetables, nuts and seeds, are good sources of fiber and are the cornerstone of the 21-Day Tummy diet.

Disaster #4: Diarrhea

Everyone has experienced diarrhea at one time or another, but some get more than their fair share. These people are all too familiar with the rush to the bathroom, the rush of the bowels. The opposite of constipation, diarrhea is runny stool. In addition to loose stool, people with diarrhea may experience cramps or abdominal pain, nausea, or dehydration.

Diarrhea can be acute or chronic. Acute diarrhea lasts approximately 1 to 2 days. Diarrhea that persists for 2 to 4 weeks is considered chronic, whether the diarrhea is mild or severe.

It's estimated that each year, U.S. adults experience 99 million episodes of acute diarrhea, resulting in about 8 million physician visits and more than 250,000 hospital admissions each year.[20] Up to 15 million Americans suffer from chronic diarrhea.[21] Worldwide, an estimated 4.5 billion people suffer from diarrhea annually.[22]

Diarrhea causes you to lose fluids at a faster rate than normal, frequently leading to dehydration. If you find yourself feeling thirsty, dizzy, or tired and/or you have dark urine or urinate less frequently, you may be experiencing the side effects of dehydration. Moderate dehydration causes you to lose strength and stamina. It's the primary cause of heat exhaustion. In its early stages, it's forgiving, but if dehydration becomes severe, it's not easy to reverse. It can affect your kidney function and cause kidney stones to develop. Severe dehydration can be serious and cause seizures, brain damage, and death. If you experience any symptoms of dehydration, have diarrhea for more than two days, have severe abdominal pain, have a fever over 102 degrees, or have black or bloody stool, see your doctor.

What Causes Diarrhea?

Acute diarrhea is usually the result of an infection. If we are infected by contaminated food, we call it food poisoning; if we're not sure what's infected us, we often blame "stomach flu," even though the influenza virus is usually not the culprit. Chronic diarrhea can also be caused infections: by bacteria (such as campylobacter, *Clostridium difficile, E. coli*, salmonella, and shigella), viruses (such as norovirus or rotavirus), or parasites (such as cryptosporidium or giardia). These infections may be accompanied by fever, bloody stool, or chills.

Noninfectious causes of chronic diarrhea are harder to diagnose, but generally diarrhea occurs when you are unable to properly digest the foods you eat. Medical conditions that affect the endocrine (hormonal) system (such as hyperthyroidism or diabetes), the pancreas (such as pancreatitis or cystic fibrosis), the immune system (such as AIDS or autoimmune disorders), and the intestines (such as ulcerative colitis or Crohn's disease)—which all play a critical part in digestion—can cause chronic diarrhea. Some cancers produce diarrhea-causing hormones. Surgery or radiation therapy in the abdominal area also causes diarrhea, as do many medications, including some antibiotics, laxatives, diuretics, chemotherapy drugs, and antacids that contain magnesium.

UPS AND DOWNS: THE THRILL (NOT) OF NAUSEA

Nausea: It's one of the symptoms we've all experienced. It can be slight and mildly unsettling, or it can be so uncomfortable and violent that it initiates a purge of stomach content. Nausea can be the result of food poisoning, food allergy, motion sickness, dehydration, disease, or even something as simple as stress. It can indicate conditions ranging from vertigo to pregnancy!

The fact that nausea is so ambiguous and can often be caused by factors unrelated to digestion is why it's not one of the digestive disorders we focused on. If you find yourself feeling nauseous or experiencing bouts of vomiting on a regular basis for more than a month, see a physician for a diagnosis.

But the most common causes of noninfectious chronic diarrhea are food intolerances. When your body lacks the enzymes to digest a food properly, or when a food irritates your stomach, you may experience diarrhea, cramps, gas, and bloating. This hypersensitivity to particular foods is an intolerance, as opposed to a food allergy, which occurs when your immune system mistakes food for an invader, triggering an inflammatory response.

The best known food intolerances, or sensitivities, are to lactose and gluten. While most people are born with the ability to digest lactose, by adulthood 75 percent of people worldwide are lactose intolerant.[23] The Center for Celiac Research at the University of Maryland estimates that approximately 18 million Americans suffer from gluten intolerance,[24] while a recent study estimates that one in every 141 Americans has celiac disease.[25] Another indicated that many cases of celiac disease go undiagnosed, but that its prevalence has risen dramatically over the past 50 years.[26] Estimates in Canada and Europe are similar.

(continued on page 68)

Weight has been a struggle for Tonya Carkeet her whole life. While she would lose a few pounds here and there, they always came back—and then some, especially after she endured a difficult pregnancy and difficult delivery of her daughter, Trista.

Tonya struggled to adjust to life as a working mom. Her weight ballooned to a high of 280 pounds, a number that hit home when she was watching a television show in which "some guys were bugging one of the characters about his weight, and it turned out I weighed more than him. It was devastating." At that weight, she says, "something always hurt." Tonya suffered from constant muscle aches, severe heartburn, diarrhea, and stomach pains, and her blood sugar was near diabetic levels.

By the time Trista turned 2, Tonya was finding it

Setting an Example by Slimming Down

exhausting to keep up with her. Plus, "Trista is the first grandbaby in the family, and everywhere we went there were always cameras. I would literally hide from them. I wondered if something were to happen to me, if Trista would even remember what I looked like or if she would be ashamed of me from the few pictures there were. I realized that I was not living the life I wanted and certainly not modeling the legacy that I wanted to pass on to my little girl."

Tonya began her weight loss journey with the Digest Diet and had lost more than 40 pounds with it when we invited her to try the 21-Day Tummy plan. Despite her success, she was nervous about giving up garlic and onions—"the things (other than butter and fat and sugar and salt) that make food taste good!" To her surprise, she loved the food: "I think the food is amazing. The meals are pretty straightforward and easy to prepare."

And after 21 days, her heartburn, diarrhea, and stomach pains were completely gone. An unexpected bonus? Her feelings of depression lifted, while her optimism, energy, and self-confidence soared. Best of all was seeing Trista learn to love new, healthy foods. "It's hard to believe I was content to live the old way for so long," Tonya says. "I feel better, I look better, and the future is much brighter."

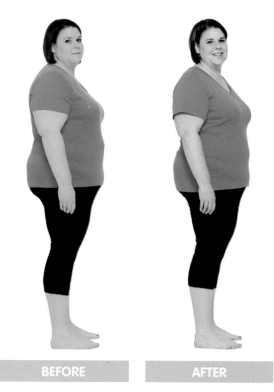

BEFORE AFTER

Tonya Carkeet

Age 32

Lost 6 POUNDS and 4 BELLY INCHES in 21 days!

Proudest accomplishments: Trimmed 4 inches from her waist; modeled healthy habits for her daughter; her digestive symptoms and feelings of depression disappeared

Favorite meal: Curried Chicken Soup

(continued from page 65)

How Can You Prevent or Treat Diarrhea?

Because the primary danger posed by diarrhea is dehydration, proper hydration is key to helping you bounce back from diarrhea. Water makes up more than two-thirds of the healthy human body. It lubricates the digestive system, as well as the joints and eyes, and flushes out waste and toxins. When the normal water content of your body is reduced, the balance of electrolytes (minerals that carry an electric charge) in your body is upset.

To treat and prevent mild to moderate dehydration, simply drink more fluids. The best choice is plain water. Liquids that contain electrolytes, such as fruit juices, sports drinks, and salty broths can help you recover fluids faster than plain water, but they can contain carb-dense sugars, belly-bloating sodium, or tummy-troubling FODMAPs.[27] (Coconut water is one exception; it can be a belly-friendly source of electrolytes.) Avoid caffeine and alcohol, which can be dehydrating.

In cases of acute diarrhea, you may resort to an over-the-counter medication like Imodium (loperamide), which slows down gut contractions and reduces the secretion of fluids in your digestive tract. Long-term use, though, can lead to constipation. Your doctor has also probably told you to try some variation of the BRAT (bananas, rice, apples, toast) diet. These bland, simple carbohydrates are easier to digest and are thought to be less likely to bother most people's stomachs. But, in fact, if your diarrhea is related to a food intolerance, bread might actually make it worse. The 21-Day Tummy diet eliminates foods you might not tolerate, but it adds back a cornucopia of delicious soothing foods, so you don't have to avoid taste and flavor in order to avoid the runs.

TUMMY **TWISTER** OR **TAMER?** Dairy Foods

I was thrilled when Kate explained that not all dairy foods have equal amounts of lactose and that even those with lactose intolerance are usually okay with small amounts of lactose; that meant I didn't have to swear off milk and other dairy foods altogether! Hard cheeses, like cheddar, Swiss, or Parmesan, for instance, generally have less than a gram of lactose per serving. And plain Greek yogurt is relatively low in lactose because more of the lactose-containing liquid whey is drained off than in regular yogurt. Processed cheeses and flavored yogurts may have milk, whey, or other milk products added back in for flavor; those can bump the lactose content up again.

Disaster #5:
Irritable Bowel Syndrome

You probably know how uncomfortable gas pain and bloating can be; perhaps you've experienced the sluggishness that comes with constipation; maybe you've done your dash to the bathroom with diarrhea. Now, imagine dealing with all three at once, all the time, and you've got irritable bowel syndrome (IBS).

A chronic digestive disorder affecting the large intestine, IBS affects up to 20 percent of Americans.[28] Canada has one of the highest rates of IBS in the world, with about 5 million people diagnosed in 2008 and 120,000 new cases each year.[29] Estimates suggest that only one in four people with IBS actually see a doctor for their symptoms—some may be too embarrassed, some may think they're normal, and others may just decide it's not worth the time to deal with. A definitive diagnosis for IBS is often difficult because the symptoms are so common and can be caused by so many diseases.

> The most common causes of noninfectious chronic diarrhea are food intolerances.

What Causes IBS?

Researchers don't really know what causes IBS, but it's clear that the nerves in the bowel appear to be extra sensitive in people who have this disorder. In IBS, your intestines can move too fast, leading to diarrhea, or too slow, contributing to constipation. And because they don't move properly, they can trap gas, causing bloating.

IBS is usually diagnosed before the age of 35, and those with a family history of IBS may be at a higher risk. Women receive the IBS diagnosis more frequently than men, but it's unclear if this is because IBS is actually more common in women or because women are more likely (four times more likely!) to report these symptoms to their doctor.[30] Given the fact that women report increased symptoms during their menstrual cycle, though, researchers do think that hormones likely play a role in IBS.

While stress does not cause IBS, it's been proven to aggravate symptoms for those who already have it. In a review of the literature, researchers at the UCLA School of Medicine found ample evidence for a link between stress and IBS. They found that individuals who experience severe traumas (such as abuse, rape, loss of a primary caregiver early in childhood) were more likely to develop functional GI disorders like IBS later in life, and that up to 40 percent of those with IBS exhibit "increased anxiety."[31] This doesn't mean that only folks who have survived a trauma suffer from IBS; even garden-variety stressors can tie your stomach in knots.

And, of course, what you eat can contribute to IBS as well. A 2009 study published in the *Journal of the American Dietetic Association* showed that for one-quarter of IBS sufferers, their symptoms were "caused or exacerbated" by eating "fermentable, poorly absorbed carbohydrates, including fructose, fructans (present in wheat and onions), sorbitol, and other sugar alcohols."[32] Sound familiar? That's right, these are all FODMAPs, which are minimized on the 21-Day Tummy plan.

How Can You Prevent and Treat IBS Symptoms?

Because the causes of IBS are unknown, treatment focuses on relieving symptoms. Among the recommendations are:

- Reduce stress.
- Increase physical activity.
- Avoid gas-producing foods.

Hopefully, these sound familiar to you by now. The 21-Day Tummy diet cuts out foods that promote gas, while the 21-Day Tummy workout includes a yoga routine that incorporates exercise and relaxation into one therapeutic session.

In addition, probiotic supplements may help. A 2013 study published in the journal *Gastroenterology* showed not only that stress upsets the balance of gut flora in a way that contributes to IBS, but also that probiotics reversed the effects, at least in mice.[33]

Luckily, research shows that IBS does not lead to other diseases; the main concern among many of those with IBS is that it greatly affects their quality of life. It ranks second in reasons why people miss work, right behind the common cold.[34] You may find it helpful to join a support group for people with IBS; look online, or ask your doctor for recommendations. Hypnotherapy can also be very effective. And, while no one solution fits everyone with IBS, the 21-Day Tummy meal plan is a safe place to start and may give you back control over your bowels and your life.

> Nerves in the bowel appear to be extra sensitive in people who have IBS.

***

Gas and bloating, heartburn and acid reflux, constipation, diarrhea, and IBS—these digestive disorders are disastrous for your waistline and your well-being in and of themselves. Now it's time to ensure that these discomforts don't develop into even more serious, or even life-threatening, diseases such as GERD, inflammatory bowel disease, or esophageal or colon cancer. The 21-Day Tummy diet offers a five-in-one solution that addresses all five issues at the same time and trims your beer (or wine) gut. The first step? Avoiding the Belly Bullies that can cause or exacerbate your tummy troubles.

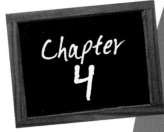

Chapter 4

Belly Bullies
That May Trouble Your Tummy

Potentially problematic food choices are all around us. I call these Belly Bullies. That's not to say that every exchange with a bully leads to tears. We can have a little bit of difficult-to-digest food here and there and our bellies will be fine, but having to endure a bully day after day will make your stomach churn, especially if you have a sensitive digestive system.

When people who are prone to gastrointestinal problems eat too many Belly Bullies, symptoms flare up. For instance, I am able to digest a glass of milk just fine, but not with a bowl of carb-dense, FODMAP-containing whole wheat cereal—it's the combination that hurts. In the 21-Day Tummy meal plan, you're going to cleanse your system of Belly Bullies. This will soothe your gut and shrink your tummy. Then, when you start to add them back in, you'll discover what your particular bullies are and how to handle them.

What Are the Belly Bullies?

Chronic inflammation and an imbalanced gut microbiome are at the root of both excess belly fat and digestive woes. Carb-dense foods are linked to both. Pro-inflammatory fats promote chronic inflammation. FODMAPs feed your gut flora, potentially throwing them out of balance; we focus on five types: lactose, fructose, fructans, galacto-oligosaccharides, and polyols.

Together, these are the Belly Bullies we minimize on the 21-Day Tummy plan. You'll see that some foods fall under more than one category; those are especially important to avoid. In this chapter, Kate and I will explain what to watch out for in each category, but first here's a quick-reference list of the top foods to dodge for the next 21 days:

1. **Carb-dense foods** (refined carbs and grains): white flour, sugar

2. **Pro-inflammatory fats** (trans fats, saturated fats, omega-6 fats): red meat, processed foods, fast food, full-fat cheese, fatty processed meats like salami and bologna

3. **High-lactose foods:** milk, regular yogurt

4. **High-fructose foods:** high-fructose corn syrup, honey, agave nectar, mangoes, apples, pears

5. **High-fructan foods:** wheat, garlic, onions and relatives (leeks, shallots), chicory root extract (inulin)

6. **High-GOS (galacto-oligosaccharide) foods:** beans/legumes, especially red kidney beans and soybeans

7. **High-polyol foods:** artificial sugars, plums, prunes, apricots, nectarines, blackberries, mushrooms, cauliflower, sugar-free mints and gum

Belly Bully #1: Carb-Dense Foods

Many foods that are carb-dense alter the balance of our gut flora, triggering an inflammatory response that can lead to both big bellies and unhappy tummies. Plus, many carb-dense foods are also high in FODMAPs (especially excess fructose and fructans). No wonder they lead the list of Belly Bullies we should avoid!

It's been pounded into the collective nutrition consciousness that whole grains are good sources of fiber and therefore important to a healthy diet and smooth digestion. But almost all grains are, by their very nature, carb-dense. The grains that we eat produce a tissue called endosperm inside their seeds. The endosperm is designed to provide concentrated nutrition in the form of starch to the plant embryos, so they are really packed with carbs.

Refined grains, which contain just the seed and endosperm, are especially carb-dense. It turns out that the carb density of muffins can lead to "muffin tops." The irony! It's pretty easy to identify these—for the next 3 weeks, ban anything made of flour (think pastries, pretzels, pizza) or with a lot of sugar (cookies, cereals, candies).

> The carb density of muffins can lead to "muffin tops." The irony!

Whole or unrefined grains include the plant embryo (called the germ) and seed coat (called the bran), which add some fiber and other ingredients. It's true that whole grains are less carb-dense and more nutritious than refined grains. But they still weigh in quite a bit higher than the 30 percent carb density we're aiming for on the 21-Day Tummy plan. The carb density of whole wheat cereal, for instance, is about 65 percent; of bran cereal, about 45 percent. So, while whole grains are a healthier choice than refined grains, eating too many of them or eating the wrong ones can lead to weight gain and bother your belly.

TUMMY **TWISTER** OR **TAMER?** Corn

Corn comes in many varieties, such as popcorn, on the cob, and in polenta. Fresh sweet corn contains two types of FODMAPs, GOS and sorbitol; this combination makes corn challenging for some people to digest. Popcorn feels like a light and healthy snack, but it's actually carb-dense (it has about 64 grams of carbs per 100 grams) and may also have trans fats added to help make it shelf stable. (Of course, topping it with salt and/or butter doesn't make it any healthier!) But whole meal cornmeal and corn tortillas seem to be better tolerated by most people so you'll see that they are used on the 21-Day Tummy meal plan. Whole grain polenta is also low in FODMAPs. As with all potentially problematic foods, you may need to experiment a little to figure out which corn products work for you. And stick with only limited quantities (up to 1 cup cooked per serving).

Adding fuel to the fire is the fact that sugar is added to many grain products, from the aforementioned cereals (even healthy whole-grain varieties) to granola bars and even to some breads. Since sugar has a carb density of 99.98 grams per 100 grams, it can make these foods more carb-dense. (Different types of sugar have slightly different carb densities, but they are all close to 100 percent.) Sugar also contributes additional calories and leads to inflammation. In a recent study of healthy young men of normal weight, those who drank sugar-sweetened beverages increased their levels of C-reactive protein, an inflammatory marker, by 60 to 109 percent (depending on the amount and type of sugar consumed).[1]

In the first phase of the 21-Day Tummy diet, Kate has taken grains off the menu entirely to let your belly settle down. But because grains and carbs have been shown to increase serotonin levels and keep mood and energy up, especially in women, she didn't want to cut them out entirely. Luckily, there are a few grains that are carb-light, so you'll see those on your Belly Buddies list in Chapter 5.

What about starchy vegetables like potatoes, corn, and winter squash? We often think of these as carbs, and many diets lump them together with grains as foods to limit. But as we saw in Chapter 2, while foods may be carb-rich, they are not necessarily carb-dense, because they contain water and other ingredients that "dilute" the carbs.

The following list is not meant to be exhaustive, but will give you an idea of the types of carb-dense foods we will avoid while on the 21-Day Tummy diet:

Bagels

Bread (including whole grain breads)

Cookies

Crackers (including whole wheat crackers and rye crispbreads)

Muffins

Pretzels

Pasta (especially if made with white flour)

Refined cereals (such as cornflakes and puffed rice)

Refined grains (such as white flour and white rice)

Rice cakes (made with white rice)

Belly Bully #2: Pro-Inflammatory Fats

Three types of dietary fat are linked with inflammation and thus pile on to our belly fat: trans fats, saturated fats, and omega-6 fats.

Trans fats, or partially hydrogenated oils, are found in many carb-dense foods such as commercially baked goods. Other packaged foods, especially those that don't need refrigeration, can be sources of trans fats since these fats are designed to help keep food from spoiling. Think microwave popcorn, sandwich cookies, and cake frosting. While I don't advocate that you go crazy counting every last gram of trans fats, there's nothing about them that helps your body in any way, so steer clear as much as possible!

> Packaged foods that don't need refrigeration are sources of trans fats.

Saturated fats are found in animal products like meat, poultry, and dairy. Think about the marbling in steaks, the greasy skin of chicken, and the richness of butter, cream, and cheese. Our bodies do use saturated fat (just as cows and chickens do) both as a source of energy and as building material for cell membranes. But we convert excess carbs in our body into saturated fatty acids for storage, so we don't really need to eat any.[2] (That's why, unlike unsaturated fats, saturated fat is not considered an "essential fatty acid.")

Because foods contain a mix of different types of fat, it's tough to cut saturated fat out of our diets completely. To do so would mean cutting out sources of healthy fats, such as those found in olives, avocados, nuts, and seeds. But since saturated fat has been implicated in heart disease, type 2 diabetes, and cancer, along with the extra weight and stomach problems that come with inflammation and microbial imbalance, it's wise to cut back on foods that are high in saturated fats.

KNOWLEDGE NIBBLES

Because fat is challenging to digest, it causes bloating. Spices, especially ginger and curcumin, help you digest fat. A 2011 study showed that spices stimulate the body to secrete more bile and also promote activity in the pancreas, both of which are required for breaking down fat.[3]

To my great dismay, that means pizza. The *Dietary Guidelines for Americans* recommends that we get no more than 10 percent of our calories from saturated fats; for most people, that translates to no more than 16 to 20 grams per day. Guess how much saturated fat is in my favorite slice of sausage pizza? Up to 10 grams! Exactly how much saturated fat you get will vary depending on the chain and the toppings you choose, but it doesn't change the fact that regular cheese and pizza are the top food sources of saturated fat in the American diet. They're followed by carb-dense grain-based desserts (good-bye, cakes), FODMAP-full dairy-based desserts (ta-ta, ice cream), and various meat-based dishes.[4]

Omega-6 fatty acids, on the other hand, are necessary for good health. And because our bodies don't make them, we need to get them from food (making them an "essential fatty acid"). The common source is vegetable oils. However, as we learned in Chapter 2, getting the right balance of omega-6 and omega-3 fatty acids is important, and unfortunately most of us have our proportions of these nutrients exactly backward. This toxic imbalance causes inflammation. Even if you don't cook with oils high in omega-6s, you may be consuming more omega-6s than you realize; most restaurant foods are cooked in these oils and many processed and packaged foods contain them. Check ingredient labels for the oils listed below.

The following list includes some of the major sources of inflammatory fats that Kate has removed from the 21-Day Tummy diet:

Trans Fats
Fast foods
Packaged foods

Omega-6 Fats
Corn oil
Grapeseed oil
Safflower oil
Soybean oil
Sunflower oil

Saturated Fats
Candy
Fatty cuts of beef
Full-fat dairy products
(such as whole milk,
butter, and cheese)
Pizza
Processed meat (such as
bacon, bologna, hot dogs,
pepperoni, salami, and
sausages)

Belly Bully #3: High-Lactose Foods

Lactose is the best known of the rapidly fermentable carbs called FODMAPs, and sadly, it's the one responsible for some of my uncomfortable days and nights. As a midwestern gal, I grew up enjoying tall glasses of milk, not to mention cheese and cream. But as I got older, I found that that same glass of milk started making my tummy grumble.

It wasn't my imagination. See, lactose is found in all types of animal milks—and yes, that includes human breast milk. Lactose is broken down in the small intestine by an enzyme called lactase. Since babies are designed to live exclusively on breast milk, it stands to reason that they need lots of lactase to digest it. Once they're weaned, they move on to eating other foods and no longer need lactase as much. So the human body is genetically programmed to reduce lactase production after that.[5] A few lucky populations, though, mostly in Europe (where dairy farming—and thus the habit of continuing to drink milk well into adulthood—started early) evolved to continue producing lactase.[6] That's why lactose intolerance is more common among Asian and African populations than Caucasians.

While you can't reprogram your genes to produce more lactase, you can recruit your friendly gut bacteria to help you digest more dairy. Some strains of bacteria, including *Bifidobacterium longum* and *Bifidobacterium animalis*, break down lactose without fermenting it, thus reducing the symptoms of excess gas or bloating.[7] You can encourage the growth of these lactose-loving bacteria by gradually building up to larger amounts of milk, or by eating yogurt with these cultures, or by taking supplements. And, of course, you can also take lactase enzyme supplements to help you manage symptoms before you eat problematic foods.

As with all FODMAPs, everyone differs in their sensitivity to lactose, but even most lactose-intolerant people can tolerate up to 4 grams of lactose per serving. Because dairy is such a good source of calcium, along with vitamins A, D, and K, and has been demonstrated to help with weight loss, we've incorporated low-lactose dairy (mostly in the form of Greek yogurt and reduced-fat cheese) throughout the 21-Day Tummy meal plan. (We also include many nondairy sources of calcium, such as kale and chia seeds.) If you're especially sensitive to lactose, you can replace these with nondairy or lactose-free substitutes, but I do urge you to try the plan as written first. Since we are taking other FODMAPs out of your diet, you may find that you can tolerate more dairy than you thought or that your symptoms were in fact not caused by lactose but by another FODMAP or combination of FODMAPs. (This is what I quickly discovered.) Conversely, even if you're pretty sure you're not lactose-intolerant, stick with lactose-free milk as called for in the plan to really clear your system of FODMAPs. You can switch back to regular milk after your 21 days.

Here's the list of high-lactose foods you should minimize while on the 21-Day Tummy plan:

Milk (includes whole, low-fat, and skim; includes goat's milk and sheep's milk)

Milk powder or milk solids

Evaporated milk

Sweetened condensed milk

Regular (non-Greek) yogurt

Soft cheeses (such as cottage cheese, crème fraîche, mascarpone, and ricotta)

Dairy-based desserts (such as ice cream, pudding, flan, crème brûlée, tiramisu, and cheesecake)

Belly Bully #4: High-Fructose Foods

Fructose occurs naturally in many foods, but these days we tend to get a lot of it in unnatural ways, thanks to the ubiquity of high-fructose corn syrup (also sometimes called corn sugar, glucose-fructose syrup, or high-fructose maize syrup). A refined sugar that's been linked with inflammation, high-fructose corn syrup has been the subject of controversy regarding its role in the current obesity epidemic. Manufacturers, who like the fact that it's cheap to make, claim that it's all natural and no different than any other type of sugar.

But foods with too much of it can contribute to gas, bloating, and diarrhea. A 2008 study in the *Journal of Clinical Gastroenterology* found that IBS patients put on a nonfructose diet experienced a significant reduction of belching, bloating, fullness, and diarrhea.[8] Some studies have also shown that high-fructose corn syrup may be associated with excess weight, especially around the middle. In a 2010 Princeton University study, for instance, rats with access to high-fructose corn syrup gained "significantly more weight" than those with access to table sugar, even though their overall caloric intake was the same.[9]

> The biggest problem with high-fructose corn syrup is how much of it we're eating.

The researchers also found that long-term consumption of high-fructose corn syrup led to abnormal increases in body fat, especially in the abdomen, and a rise in triglycerides, which are associated with high cholesterol and heart disease. "When rats are drinking high-fructose corn syrup at levels well below those in soda pop," said Bart Hoebel, one of the study's authors, "they're becoming obese, every single one. . . . Even when rats are fed a high-fat diet, you don't see this."

In another study of 32 overweight or obese people, those who consumed fructose gained more dreaded belly fat than those who had similar amounts of glucose. Their triglyceride, blood sugar, and insulin levels all increased, as well.[10]

In addition, growing evidence points to the fact that the body metabolizes glucose and fructose differently. Every cell in the body metabolizes glucose, whereas only the liver metabolizes fructose. This means that drinks and food containing high amounts of fructose hit the liver faster. Research in lab rats has shown that the larger the amount of fructose and the faster it hits the liver, the more likely the liver is to turn the fructose into fat.[11] That's bad in and of itself, but even worse, this liver response can lead to insulin resistance, which causes the body to secrete more insulin than necessary when you eat food, making your blood sugar levels rise. What comes next? Diabetes.

But the biggest problem with high-fructose corn syrup is probably just how much of it we're eating. It's used in sodas, juices, cereals, yogurts, ice pops, salad dressings, and condiments, and even in things we don't think of as sweet, such as bread, lunch meats, and soups. The average North American consumes almost 47 pounds of the stuff per year (and that's on top of the 41-plus pounds of table sugar we eat per year)![12]

In addition to its impact on our waistline, fructose is often incompletely absorbed by our GI system. This is called fructose malabsorption, and there are a number of ways it can occur. Sometimes bacteria in our small intestine get to the fructose before it's efficiently digested. Some of us don't have enough of the proteins that transport fructose across the intestinal lining. And if food moves too quickly through the digestive tract, there isn't enough time for fructose to be absorbed by our body. As with many tummy issues, some people are better able to absorb fructose than others; about one in three people are estimated to suffer from fructose malabsorption, which can lead to gas, bloating, diarrhea, and other digestive symptoms.[13] (This is me!)

When fructose is consumed together with glucose, it is able to hitch a ride with glucose through the intestinal lining. In those cases, it is better absorbed and doesn't cause digestive problems. So foods that have a balanced fructose-to-glucose ratio are fine to eat, but, as we cleanse our systems on the 21-Day Tummy diet, we want to avoid or limit the foods that are higher in fructose than in glucose (and it's not just high-fructose corn syrup). After you assess your sensitivity to excess fructose, you may (or may not) want to reintroduce them to your diet in limited quantities. Here's a list of some high-fructose foods to steer clear of:

DARN YOU, AGAVE!

We're trained to think that if something is "natural," it's healthy. Well, not only is this not always true, but natural foods that are healthy for some people aren't healthy for others. Case in point? Agave! This southwestern plant is the source of the latest "wonder food," agave nectar. It's also used to make tequila. Sounds fun, right? Well, not for me. I once sweetened my tea with agave nectar, thinking it healthier than honey, and was in so much pain I had to leave work early! Agave is more than 80 percent fructose, which can irritate the GI tract.

Fruits	Vegetables	Sweeteners
Apples	Asparagus	Agave nectar
Cherries	Artichokes	High-fructose
Mangoes	Fava beans	corn syrup
Pears	Sugar snap peas	Fruit juice
Watermelon		concentrate
		Honey

Belly Bully #5: High-Fructan Foods

Fructans are made up mostly of fructose molecules, usually with a glucose molecule tacked on at the end. Since, as we know, an excess of fructose is a problem for many people with sensitive tummies, it shouldn't come as any surprise that fructans can be a problem, too. In fact, we humans lack the enzymes to break down fructans, so no one is able to truly digest them.

Fructans are a type of fiber and, as such, can be very beneficial to your digestion and your overall health. But because fibers are, by definition, undigestible by the human body, they cause flatulence to varying degrees (depending on the type of fiber and the bacteria in your gut). Fructans seem to cause more symptoms than most, but that may simply be because we tend to eat more of them than of other types of fiber; fructans are found in a wide variety of foods, most notably wheat.

Once touted as a healthy source of complex carbohydrates and fiber, wheat has fallen out of favor, largely because of the growing awareness of gluten intolerance and celiac disease. Beyond that, wheat is now being blamed for everything from wrinkles to heart disease, and we're now seeing that many people have a difficult time digesting it. These people end up in worse shape than when their big problem was that they didn't get enough fiber.

Onions and garlic and their relatives are another major source of fructans in our food supply. Many of our testers found that cooking without onions and garlic was one of the biggest adjustments on the plan. Even if you're not a big onion or garlic fan, most commercially prepared spice mixes, salad dressings, and sauces contain onion or garlic, so it's hard to dodge them. In Chapter 7, we'll show you how you can get the flavor of onions or garlic without the belly grumbles.

Another hidden source of fructans? Take a look at the ingredients list of any products touted as "high-fiber," like cereals or breads. Then check out the ingredients of "reduced-fat" foods, like yogurts or even ice creams. Chances are you'll find chicory root extract, sometimes also listed as inulin or FOS (fructo-oligosaccharide). Inulin tastes slightly sweet so it allows food manufacturers to reduce the amount of other sugars they use; it also has a similar mouthfeel to fat so manufacturers use it as a fat substitute. At the same time, it allows them to claim a higher fiber content. To avoid this rapidly fermentable sugar, stick to foods naturally high in fiber.

Here's a list of high-fructan foods Kate has minimized on the 21-Day Tummy plan:

> **TUMMY TWISTER OR TAMER? Watermelon**
>
> This lovely summer treat isn't as harmless as all the water it contains. Watermelon is high in fructose, fructans, and polyols. Remember, the more the FODMAPs, the more potential for tummy trouble. Did you grow up hearing that if you ate watermelon seeds, you'd grow a watermelon in your stomach? That doesn't happen, of course, but watermelon can certainly cause other digestive problems if you're sensitive to FODMAPs.

Fruits
Nectarines
Persimmons
Watermelon
White peaches

Grains
Barley
Rye
Wheat

Vegetables
Artichokes
Garlic
Onions
Leeks (white part)
Scallions (white part)
Shallots

Nuts
Cashews
Pistachios

Legumes
Black beans
Black-eyed peas
Kidney beans
Lima beans
Soybeans

Additives
Inulin (also called
   chicory root extract)
FOS (fructo-
   oligosaccharides)

(continued on page 88)

Jonathan Bigham had always been trim and fit. But, he noted, "since I turned 40, I've been gaining weight only in the middle, and no matter how far I'd run or how many laps I'd do in the pool, nothing worked." Until the 21-Day Tummy plan, that is. After the plan, he crows, "I feel like I stand taller. I fit into pants that didn't fit 3 weeks ago. I've moved my belt notch back to where it used to be a couple months ago."

And he was happily surprised at "how easy it was to actually be able to cook all my meals. And that it didn't take a huge amount of time." He was even able to stick to the plan during his family vacation to Disney World, where he toted his own belly-

He Kicked a 6-Bottle-a-Day Soda Habit

friendly snacks and scouted out restaurant meals that would make his tummy happy in "the happiest place on Earth."

It helped that his energy levels skyrocketed on the plan. "Two weeks into the plan and I've been waking up without the need for an alarm all week." He also found that vigorous activities such as his regular runs became easier, and his usual bouts of diarrhea and acid reflux completely disappeared. "I no longer dread having to walk the dog every morning," he says, "and I'm less anxious about looking older than my age or having clothes that are too tight and uncomfortable."

But perhaps the biggest surprise for Jonathan? "Three weeks ago, I'd have bet $1,000 that I would never be able to go without diet sodas," he confesses. "I used to drink at least six 20-ounce bottles of diet soda every day. It was just a habit. But I don't crave it anymore. I haven't really missed it. Just give me a water, I'm good." With that change, he's even saving money on the 21-Day Tummy plan! And he's looking ahead to "the next three weeks and beyond."

Having already introduced his family to the delicious 21-Day Tummy recipes, he's looking forward to helping his wife, who was inspired by his success, to try the plan herself.

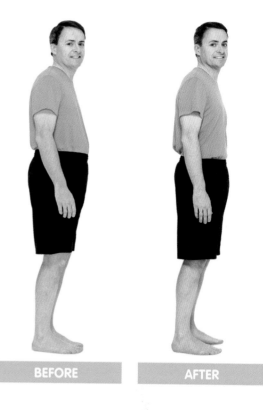

BEFORE   AFTER

Jonathan Bigham

Age 43

Lost 7½ POUNDS and 1 BELLY INCH in 21 days!

Proudest accomplishments: Kicking his diet soda addiction; losing his middle-age spread

Favorite meals: Tomato-Ginger Flank Steak; Berry Good Belly Soother Smoothie

(continued from page 85)

Belly Bully #6: High-GOS Foods

Beans contain chains of sugars called galacto-oligosaccharides. Not only do humans have a hard time saying "galacto-oligosaccharides" (hence my favorite new acronym, GOS), we also have a hard time digesting them. Humans lack the enzymes to break the chains, therefore, beans become food for gut bacteria. When the gut bacteria eat the undigested fiber in beans, they produce gas. Therein is why beans have a well-deserved reputation for contributing to gas and bloating.

Pretty much every type of bean is high in GOS, but you'll see that we've allowed a limited amount of a few of the least offensive (chickpeas, snow peas, green peas) so that you can get the benefit of the fiber without the gassiness. In addition, some nuts are also high in GOS. Here are the ones you should avoid altogether during the 21-Day Tummy plan (again, you'll have the option of adding them back in to your diet after you've settled your stomach):

TUMMY **TWISTER** OR **TAMER?** Soy Foods

Whole soybeans (often sold as edamame), like other beans, are a source of GOS. But tofu, also called bean curd, is made by coagulating soy milk with salts or acids and then pressing the resulting curds together. This process allows the troublesome GOS fibers to drain off into the liquid portion that is discarded, so tofu usually is well tolerated. Tempeh is made by fermenting soybeans; the bacteria used to make it help break down some of the GOS before you eat it, so it's also usually safe for your tummy. What about soy milk? It depends. If soy milk is made with only soybean isolates or soy protein, then it should be low in FODMAPs. Soy milk made with whole soybeans is likely a source of GOS, making soy milk a gassy beverage for some, so read the ingredients.

Beans
Adzuki beans
Black beans
Butter beans
Cannellini beans
Fava beans
Great northern
  beans
Kidney beans
Lima beans
Pinto beans
Mung beans (but
  bean sprouts are
  okay)
Navy beans
Soybeans (but tofu
  and tempeh are
  okay)

Nuts
Cashews
Pistachios

Belly Bully #7: High-Polyol Foods

Polyols are often called sugar alcohols because their chemical structure looks partly like sugar and partly like alcohol. In fact, they are neither sugar nor alcohol but, like their namesakes, they are big trouble. I think of sugar alcohols as "sugar fake, bellyache" because numerous studies have linked sugar substitutes to digestive problems.

Our cells are not able to actively transport sugar alcohols through the cell membrane, so they are left to "passively diffuse" through the digestive system. This means they hang around for a long time and are usually incompletely absorbed. That's why we don't get many calories (i.e., energy) from them; this, in turn, is why they are frequently used as sugar substitutes. But our gut bacteria have no problem fermenting sugar alcohols, and that leads to abdominal distress.[14]

Most people are unaffected by sugar alcohols because most foods don't have that much of them. But if you go for a lot of sugar-free foods because you're trying to lose weight, you may easily be eating enough sugar alcohol to cause excessive flatulence, gas pain, or diarrhea. Because the relative sweetness in most sugar alcohols is less than that of sugar, most sugar-free products use a lot of them.

Because polyols are the main component in sugar substitutes, we tend to think of them as fake, but some sugar alcohols occur naturally in foods. For instance, sorbitol, a common sugar alcohol, is found in blackberries and stone fruits such as peaches, plums, apricots, cherries, and even avocados. Snow peas add a nice crunch to Asian stir-fries but also contain fructans and GOS plus a big dose of mannitol, another naturally occurring sugar alcohol.

For the duration of the 21-Day Tummy plan, Kate has removed all high-polyol foods. After your tummy has settled down, you may

> ## TUMMY **TWISTER** OR **TAMER?** Blackberries
>
> Strawberries, blueberries, blackberries—which is the odd one out here? Blackberries, while rich in antioxidants, are also rich in polyols, which can cause some real problems if your stomach is sensitive to them.

choose to add back many of these yummy real foods (though perhaps in smaller quantities than you enjoyed them before). Remember, even though these fruits and vegetables contain FOD-MAPs, they are healthy. But I would recommend that you steer clear of artificial sweeteners even if you discover that you aren't sensitive to polyols. They may ultimately undermine your weight loss efforts, and they don't offer any benefits to your body.

Here, the high-polyol foods Kate has eliminated on the 21-Day Tummy plan:

Fruits	Vegetables	Artificial Sweeteners/ Additives
Apples	Cauliflower	
Apricots	Mushrooms	Isomalt
Blackberries	Snow peas	Mannitol
Cherries		Maltitol
Nectarines	Sugar-Free Foods	Maltitol
Peaches	Candy	Polydextrose
Pears	Gums	Sorbitol
Plums	Mints	Xylitol
Prunes		
Watermelon		

***

You've probably noticed that FODMAPs exist in foods that are extremely different from each other. Who would have thought that garlic and sugar-free gum would have similar consequences? But thanks to the quirks of our digestive system, both can cause gas, bloating, and other GI issues—as can a whole host of otherwise healthy foods. Add in the carb-dense foods and pro-inflammatory fats you need to beware of, and it can feel like you're left with even less to eat than on low-carb or low-fat diets.

But I'm happy to report that that's not true—in fact, the 21-Day Tummy plan has opened my palate to a wide range of foods I'd never liked before but now love (like fish, parsnips, and turnips). Kate has wisely replaced the important nutrients found in the healthy (but distressing) foods so we're not missing out on vital nutrients. Let me introduce you to the amazingly yummy, fat-shrinking, tummy-soothing Belly Buddies!

Belly Buddies
That Soothe and Shrink Your Stomach

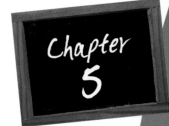

Chapter
5

Enough about forbidden foods. Let's talk about all the stuff we can eat on the 21-Day Tummy plan!

I'm not just talking about foods that are low in the refined carbs, inflammatory fats, and FODMAPs that can cause gastrointestinal upset. We've put the spotlight on foods that do double duty! A mix of antioxidant-rich fruits and vegetables, lean protein, and healthy fats, our Belly Buddies actively combat the twin evils of inflammation and imbalanced gut flora—which means they both soothe and shrink your belly. They also provide balanced nutrition to support general good health.

The best part? They're delicious! And don't worry, you won't have to make a special trip to a gourmet grocery to find them; I bet most of them are already in your fridge.

What Are the Belly Buddies?

The stars of the 21-Day Tummy diet, Belly Buddy foods are carb-light and low in FODMAPs. In order to help us lose weight while at the same time keeping our digestive system humming, they also feature these stomach-soothing ingredients:

- **Fiber** is key to keeping things moving in our digestive tract. But not just any fiber will do. Certain types of fiber are rapidly fermentable and can therefore knock our GI system for a loop, so we focus on foods that contain insoluble fiber and select soluble fibers.

- **Magnesium** is a mineral that your cells need to make energy and your muscles need to relax; a deficiency in this critical nutrient has been strongly associated with increased inflammation.[1]

- **Anti-inflammatory fats,** including MUFAs and omega-3s, help keep inflammation at bay, as their name implies. Some also do a good job of targeting the fat in and around your belly.

PACKING LUNCHES CAN HELP YOU LOSE WEIGHT AND SAVE CASH

I can't remember the last time I scheduled a business lunch. I've always preferred breakfast (faster) or dinner (more fun!). For 25 years, I've been a lunch packer. Dining out during the workday is time-consuming and expensive and, since restaurant food is often filled with dense carbs, pro-inflammatory fats, and FODMAPs, it's not good for your tummy, either.

That's why we made our 21-Day Tummy lunches quick to make and easy to pack. Brown bagging it may not look glamorous, but it gives you more control, saves money, and keeps your waistline in check. Bringing a lunch doesn't mean forsaking a break. If it's a nice day, eat in a nearby park or a bench outside your workplace. Or walk down the hall and invite a coworker to join you.

In this chapter, Kate and I will describe each Belly Buddy category in more detail, but here's a quick-reference list.

1. **High-fiber and antioxidant-rich vegetables,** especially kale, Swiss chard, and spinach; also green beans, bean sprouts, bok choy, carrots, cucumbers, eggplant, endive, lettuce, parsnips, turnips, tomatoes, zucchini, and potatoes

2. **Balanced-fructose fruits,** especially bananas and blueberries; also grapes, oranges, strawberries, kiwis, pineapple, papaya, cantaloupe, honeydew, raspberries, and star fruit

3. **Low-FODMAP, high-fiber grains,** especially oats, brown rice, and quinoa; also buckwheat, polenta, and rice bran

4. **Nuts and nut butters,** especially peanuts and walnuts

5. **Seeds,** especially chia, pumpkin, and flax

6. **Healthy fats** (omega-3s, MUFAs): salmon, mackerel, tuna, herring, sardines, flaxseed, olive oil, canola oil, and olives

7. **Lean protein:** fish and seafood, poultry, lean cuts of beef and pork, eggs

8. **Greek yogurt**

9. **Coconut milk**

10. **Ginger**

11. **Turmeric**

12. **Maple syrup**

Belly Buddy #1: High-Fiber and Antioxidant-Rich Vegetables

All veggies are good for you. They are high in vitamins, minerals, phytonutrients, antioxidants, and fiber. And they are generally low in calories and low in fat. But certain varieties do contain FODMAPS that are difficult for some people to digest. Our plan focuses only on vegetables that are low in FODMAPs, with special attention on those rich in anti-inflammatory magnesium and other important minerals.

Standouts in this category are leafy green vegetables, especially kale, Swiss chard, and spinach.

Kale contains more than 45 different antioxidants, many with anti-inflammatory properties. A 1-cup serving of cooked kale, for instance, contains almost a full day's supply of beta-carotene, a precursor of vitamin A, which may inhibit the formation of pro-inflammatory immune cells while promoting the production of anti-inflammatory immune cells.[2] Kale is also rich in vitamin C, which not only combats inflammation but trimmed body mass and waist circumference in a study of 20 obese adults.[3] And kale is one of the best nondairy sources of calcium; we absorb the type of calcium in kale better than the types in spinach or other leafy greens.[4] Since research continues to pile up showing that calcium aids in weight loss—and since we're reducing FODMAP-rich dairy on the 21-Day Tummy plan—kale has become my new best buddy.

As for Swiss chard, it contains a total rock star called syringic acid. Syringic acid has received special attention in recent research because of its ability to help stabilize blood sugar.[5] This helps prevent the cravings that lead us to overeat and gain weight. Swiss chard is also rich in magnesium; just one cup of cooked chard contains 150 milligrams of magnesium, almost half your daily recommended allowance.

Spinach is also superhigh in magnesium, with 157 milligrams per cup when it's cooked. (While a little magnesium is lost when you cook greens, we prefer to heat them since you eat more because they've wilted down.) It's also chock-full of anti-inflammatory antioxidants that help protect our eyes, skin, bones, and immunity.

Here's a complete list of all the Belly Buddy vegetables that help slim and calm your tummy:

Arugula
Bean sprouts
Bell peppers (all varieties, including green, red, yellow, and orange)
Bok choy
Cabbage (red and green only; savoy and napa are limited)
Celeriac
Celery root
Cucumbers
Eggplant
Green beans
Lettuce (all varieties, including endive, iceberg, and romaine)

Parsnips
Potatoes (including red and white)
Okra
Radishes
Summer squash (all varieties, including pattypan, yellow, and zucchini)
Sweet potatoes (up to ½ cup per serving)
Tomatoes
Turnips
Water chestnuts
Watercress

Belly Buddy #2:
Balanced-Fructose Fruits

Some diet plans forbid fruit because it's high in sugars. But because nature's own desserts are also bursting with anti-oxidants, fiber, and other healthful ingredients, Kate and I aren't willing to put fruit in the same category as, say, fudge brownies. That said, some fruits are better for our tummies than others. On the 21-Day Tummy plan, Kate has included fruits with a balanced glucose-to-fructose ratio, which may be easier on your digestive tract than fruits with excess fructose. Luckily, many refreshing choices fall into this category. The best? Bananas and blueberries.

> Blueberries regularly make the lists of healthiest foods, no matter what criteria list makers use.

Bananas! Oh what a joy it's been to work this high-potassium fruit back into my diet after years of hearing it was a high-calorie option, too starchy and too sweet to be part of a lean diet. But, like potatoes, bananas are actually carb-light and packed with filling fiber. They are also rich in anti-inflammatory magnesium, as well as vitamin B6 (which helps even out blood sugar) and the aforementioned potassium (which contributes to lower blood pressure).

Now I eat bananas all the time! I especially love their convenience: Stick one in your purse, or keep a few at your desk. With a to-go packet of peanut butter, they also make a great snack after a workout or on a long flight. Bananas are also the base for my family's favorite morning smoothie combo (banana with a hint of cocoa and pumpkin seeds).

As for blueberries, they're small, delish, and perhaps the only naturally blue food. Blueberries regularly make the lists of "superfoods" or "healthiest foods," no matter what criteria the list makers use. Low in fat and high in fiber, blueberries are filling and relieve constipation. But what really makes these tiny fruits stand out is the dizzying list of phytonutrients they contain, including anti-inflammatory antho-cyanins, tannins, and other antioxidants that destroy the free radicals associated with everything from wrinkles to colon cancer. The antioxidants also help improve memory while combating many of the problems associated with aging, such as Alzheimer's.

Here's a complete list of the Belly Buddy fruits with a good balance of fructose to glucose:

Bananas
Blueberries
Cantaloupe
Cranberries
Grapes
Honeydew
Kiwis
Lemons

Limes
Oranges
Pineapple
Papaya
Raspberries
Star fruit
Strawberries

Belly Buddy #3: Low-FODMAP Grains

Sadly, almost all grains are carb-dense and therefore may be bad for your tummy, especially in the quantities we're used to eating them. Many, like wheat, are also high in FODMAPs. But since grains are such amazing (and delicious!) sources of belly-friendly fiber, Kate wanted to include as many as possible on the 21-Day Tummy plan. I was thrilled when Kate assured me that some low-FODMAP, high-fiber grains are also relatively carb-light.

Quinoa (pronounced KEEN-wah) has long been a favorite of mine. Slightly nutty and chewy, quinoa is actually not a true grain but more closely related to beets and spinach. It contains just 21 grams of carbs per 100 grams, making it truly carb-light. Quinoa is also high in fiber and protein, both of which make it a satisfying superfood. In fact, along with soy, quinoa is one of the few plant-based complete proteins (meaning it provides our body with all of the amino acids it needs to function). It's also naturally gluten free and contains thiamin, vitamin B6, iron, folate, zinc, potassium, and selenium, as well as anti-inflammatory magnesium. All these nutrients plus 5 grams of fiber in one cup (cooked), and for only 220 calories! Quinoa is usually beige or tan, but I like the red and black forms as well, all equally good for your tummy.

Oats are another high-fiber favorite that's relatively carb-light. According to a 2012 study, oats contain a type of sugar called beta-glucans, which prove to be good for appetite control, glucose control, and gut microbiota composition.[6] In a study of more than 200 adults, eating a whole grain oat cereal once a day for 12 weeks decreased waist circumference by more than an inch.[7] Oats are also a source of magnesium. Depending on how they're processed, though, some types of oat products may contain added sugars or FODMAPs. Stick with whole oats or oat bran, which are good sources of fiber, protein, essential fatty acids, and vitamins.

Brown rice, meanwhile, is high in fiber and also contains significant amounts of anti-inflammatory magnesium. And, because rice tends to be easy for most people to digest, doctors usually recommend it to people with GI issues as part of the belly-soothing BRAT (bananas, rice, apples, toast) diet.

You can find these high-fiber, low-FODMAP grains in the later phases of the 21-Day Tummy plan:

Brown rice	Polenta
Buckwheat	Quinoa
Oat bran	Rice bran
Oats (whole)	

Belly Buddy #4:
Nuts and Nut Butters

Nuts are concentrated nutrition, with protein, unsaturated fats, dietary fiber, vitamins, and minerals all jammed into a tiny, portable, and delicious package. The mix of protein, fat, and fiber makes nuts a great source of sustained energy. In one Purdue University study, researchers found that people who ate peanuts or peanut butter for a snack stayed satisfied for 2½ hours, while people who ate other snacks got hungry again within just half an hour.[8] Nuts are also great sources of monounsaturated fatty acids, which have been shown to target visceral fat.

Because they are relatively high in calories and may contain some FODMAPs, though, don't go too "nuts" for them. When buying nut butters, get the all-natural types that don't have hydrogenated fats. If the contents look like they need a good stir, it's probably a natural product (the oil separates in natural products) and that's a good thing. You can also make nut butters very easily at home. It's as simple as putting nuts and a little salt in a food processor and blending until it's the texture you want. If you like it a little runnier, add some olive oil.

> ### TUMMY **TWISTER** OR **TAMER?**
> ### Pistachios, Cashews, Hazelnuts, and Almonds
>
> Most nuts are good for your tummy, but pistachios and cashews are high in fructans and GOS, both FODMAPs. Hazelnuts and almonds are a little higher in FODMAPs than some other nuts so eat them in limited quantities (10 nuts or 1 tablespoon nut butter per serving). Steer clear of almond milk, though, which is made with large amounts of almonds.

Peanuts, in particular, are a great choice because they are also high in anti-inflammatory magnesium; one ounce of contains 50 milligrams. Go unsalted to avoid any extra bloat-inducing sodium. Be careful of dry-roasted peanuts. They often contain dried onion and garlic, which are concentrated sources of fructans; also, they may be contaminated with gluten in the processing plant. Walnuts are the only nuts with a significant amount of anti-inflammatory omega-3 fats; ¼ cup provides 2.5 grams. Peanuts and walnuts, along with pecans, are the nuts lowest in FODMAPs.

Here's a list of nuts that are low in FODMAPs; enjoy a handful of any of these crunchy treats on the 21-Day Tummy plan:

Almonds (up to 10 almonds per serving)	Peanuts
	Pecans
Hazelnuts (up to 10 hazelnuts per serving)	Pine nuts
	Walnuts
Macadamia nuts	

Belly Buddy #5: Seeds

Like nuts, seeds are great sources of low-fermentable fiber and anti-inflammatory fats along with satiating protein. They are also rich in antioxidants that can protect against cell damage from chronic inflammation.

Chia, pumpkin, and flaxseeds, for instance, all contain anti-inflammatory magnesium and healthy omega-3 fatty acids. Chia seeds, in addition, provide calcium (1 ounce of chia seeds has more calcium than half a glass of milk!). This is particularly good for people who are lactose-intolerant and don't get enough calcium through dairy. And with 5 grams of fiber in just one tablespoon, they're a marvelous carb-light, low-FODMAP source of this important nutrient.

Pumpkin seeds are high in glutamate, a substance that helps your body manufacture GABA, a brain chemical that reduces stress. Pumpkin seeds are good both raw and roasted. Next time you carve a pumpkin, scoop out the seeds. It takes some time to separate them from all the gook, but after that they just need a good rinse. Spread them on an oiled cookie sheet, sprinkle with salt, and bake in a preheated oven at 325 degrees Fahrenheit until they're golden brown. (This can take anywhere from 5 to 20 minutes, depending on how big the seeds are.) You may want to flip the halfway through the cook time. Raw or baked, they're chewy, delicious, and a lot healthier than a bag of chips. You can eat the shells, which add fiber, or crack them open to get to the meaty seed inside.

Another option is to buy de-shelled pumpkin seeds (called pepitas) and toss them into your smoothie or onto your oats in the morning. I much prefer this route. All the taste, none of the work!

Flaxseeds contain lignans, a type of phytochemical that may help protect against certain cancers. Whole flaxseeds pass through your body undigested, so be sure to either buy ground flaxseeds or grind your own with a coffee grinder. Flaxseed oil can also be a good choice, though it doesn't have the fiber.

Here's a list of all the seeds that give you a flatter and happier belly:

Chia seeds
Flax seeds
Pumpkin seeds
Sesame seeds
Sunflower seeds

Belly Buddy #6: Healthy Fats

When I was first starting out as a health journalist, most people—even most doctors—thought fat was inherently bad. Thanks to my job, I was lucky enough to learn early on about the research then just emerging about how some types of fat are really our friends. Since then, the science has continued to pile up, and most of it points to two types of fats in particular that we should eat more of: omega-3 fatty acids and monounsaturated fatty acids.

> I was lucky to learn early on about how some types of fat are really our friends.

You'll usually hear omega-3 fatty acids talked about in conjunction with omega-6 fatty acids, and that's because the two work together to regulate inflammation, among other things. Both omega-3s and omega-6s are precursors of fats called eicosanoids. The eicosanoids from omega-6s trigger inflammatory responses, while the eicosanoids from omega-3s stop them. So when the number of eicosanoids from omega-3s increases, the incidence of chronic diseases that have an inflammatory component (including inflammatory bowel disease, cardiovascular disease, and rheumatoid arthritis) drops.[9]

There are three types of omega-3 fatty acids: alpha-linolenic acid (ALA), eicosapentaenoic acid (EPA), and docosahexaenoic acid (DHA). EPA and DHA are the eicosanoids that are responsible for stopping inflammation, so they're the ones we really want. We get EPA and DHA mostly from fish, while ALA can be found in some plant oils, like flaxseed oil and walnut oil. Our bodies can make a limited amount of EPA and DHA from ALA, but it's generally not enough—which is why so many nutritionists tell you it's important to eat fish!

Monounsaturated fatty acids, otherwise known as MUFAs (pronounced MOO-fahs), are my favorites. Low levels of MUFAs have been found in people with inflammatory bowel disease, suggesting that MUFAs may lower intestinal inflammation.[10] They may also reduce "bad" cholesterol levels and maintain or increase "good" cholesterol. Best of all, they actually target dangerous visceral belly fat. A 2007 study at the Reina Sofia University Hospital in Spain observed a group of overweight individuals who were put on different diets. While they all ate the same number of calories per day, the group that had the most MUFAs lost the most belly fat.[11]

Plus, MUFAs can help us feel full (in a good way, not a bloated sense). In a 2012 German study, participants who ate olive oil yogurt reported the highest level of satisfaction and had higher levels of serotonin, a marker of satiety, in their blood. Bonus: No one in this group gained weight or body fat.[12]

Just remember that because fats are high in calories (and a few of these foods, like avacados, contain moderate amounts of FODMAPs), you'll want to keep servings relatively small.

Here's a list of some of the best sources of healthy fats:

Omega-3 Fatty Acids	MUFAs
Salmon	Avocados (up to ⅛ avocado per serving)
Tuna	
Herring	Nuts and seeds
Mackerel	Dark chocolate
Sardines	Olives and olive oil
Flaxseeds and flaxseed oil	Safflower oil
Walnuts and walnut oil	Sunflower oil
Rapeseed (canola) oil	Sesame oil
Soybean oil	

Belly Buddy #7: Lean Protein

Most of the debate about low-carb diets has been, appropriately enough, about the carbohydrates. But it turns out the secret to low-carb weight loss may not be the carbs at all, but rather what you replace them with. Most low-carb diets also happen to be high protein, and it may be the protein that is really helping those dieters lose weight. In one recent study of 130 overweight middle-age men and women, those who ate a high-protein diet lost more body fat than those following a high-carb diet.[13]

VEGETARIANS WELCOME HERE

Vegetarians are used to making substitutions at restaurants, at holiday meals, and in their own cooking. Some diets, however, make it almost impossible. Take for instance, diets that have animal protein as a majority of calories consumed. The 21-Day Tummy diet, however, makes it easy. Consider these tactics:

- Replace meat with tofu, tempeh, or eggs. You can also include small amounts of canned lentils or chickpeas (½ cup per serving of lentils, ¼ cup per serving of chickpeas). Lentils and chickpeas have fewer FODMAPs than other legumes, and canned beans in general have fewer fermentable sugars than dried beans. Rinse canned beans before you use them to further reduce fermentable sugars, as well as to lower bloat-inducing sodium.

- To get enough protein, consider higher-protein grains such as quinoa, polenta, or roasted buckwheat where recipes call for rice.

- Top salad with small amounts of reduced-fat cheese for protein.

Protein has been shown to help you feel full longer, so you end up eating less throughout the day.[14] In addition, if you're exercising to burn calories as well as dieting to restrict them, eating protein provides your body with the building blocks to create muscle during your workouts. Since your muscles burn calories even while you're at rest, the more muscle you have, the more calories you burn. Plus, those muscles give us the toned tummy we really want.

Protein is by nature carb-light and usually doesn't pose any problems to digestion (gluten, a protein found in wheat, being a notable exception). It's important to choose lean protein sources, though; many sources of protein contain a lot of pro-inflammatory saturated fat. Here are some examples of lean protein:

Eggs

Fish (especially those high in omega-3 fats, as listed on page 105)

Lean cuts of beef (such as flank steak, London broil, and tenderloin)

Lean cuts of pork (such as center cut chops and tenderloin)

Poultry (such as skinless white meat chicken and turkey)

Seafood (shellfish such as shrimp, crabs, and lobster; mollusks such as mussels, oysters, and clams)

Tofu

Tempeh

Belly Buddy #8: Greek Yogurt

All yogurts are good sources of calcium, protein, potassium, zinc, and vitamins B6 and B12. In a 12-week study, researchers at the University of Tennessee, in Knoxville, showed that participants who replaced some foods with yogurt lost more body fat and had a "markedly greater reduction in waist circumference" with "trunk [abdominal] fat loss augmented by

81% in the yogurt versus the control group."[15] Plus, of course, most yogurts have probiotic effects on the digestive system.

Greek yogurt, however, has twice the protein content of regular yogurts and is lower in lactose, a plus for anyone who might be lactose-intolerant. That's why we made it the base of our Belly Soother Smoothie. It also makes an easy, filling snack on its own and can stand in for fattening cream in many recipes.

Belly Buddy #9: Coconut Milk

Coconut products have been getting a lot of good press lately, and for good reason. This tropical fruit is rich in vitamins and minerals, along with a couple of nutrients of particular interest to those of us with tummy issues: medium-chain triglycerides and lauric acid.

Most fats are long-chain fats—and as you might imagine, the longer the chain, the longer it takes for your body to break it down to digest. That's why fats tend to linger the longest in our digestive system, which can sometimes lead to problems. More than half the fats in coconuts, though, are medium-chain triglycerides (MCTs), which are more easily digested and therefore less likely to get stored as body fat.

Lauric acid is one of these MCTs, and one that is known to have antibacterial effects.[16] While more research needs to be done, it has been suggested that, unlike antibiotics that kill both good and bad bacteria simultaneously, lauric acid is more selective and does not appear to have an adverse effect on probiotic bacteria—which could, of course, help to right any imbalances in our gut microbiome.[17]

We've zeroed in on coconut milk here as a Belly Buddy because it's a great lactose-free alternative to regular milk, providing an excellent mix of fat, vitamin E, and many other nutrients. Made by mixing coconut juice with coconut meat, then pressing it to expel the milk, coconut milk can help

(continued on page 110)

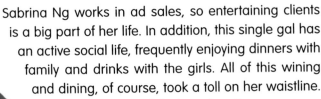

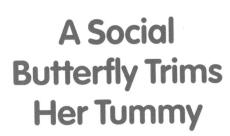

Sabrina Ng works in ad sales, so entertaining clients is a big part of her life. In addition, this single gal has an active social life, frequently enjoying dinners with family and drinks with the girls. All of this wining and dining, of course, took a toll on her waistline. And while her digestive symptoms weren't severe, they were frequent enough to be bothersome: Sabrina suffered from regular abdominal cramps, gas, bloating, diarrhea, nausea, and acid reflux.

Even though she was ready to make a change, when she first learned what she would need to do on the 21-Day Tummy diet, she was skeptical. With Chinese New Year's coming up the weekend she planned to start,

A Social Butterfly Trims Her Tummy

she fretted about how to tell her family she couldn't feast with them. Then there was Valentine's Day, when she had to dodge all the candy in the office. And the all-inclusive bachelorette party in the Bahamas, where she knew she would want to "get her money's worth" of food and drink.

For Sabrina, doing her belly good meant rethinking what it meant to have a good time. It also meant being open to trying new foods and new ways of cooking, as well as learning what appropriate portions were for some of her old favorites. Having never stuck to a strict meal plan before, she found the 21-day plan a challenge at first, but a worthwhile one. "It works!" she exclaims. "I feel so much less bloated after this diet. I love the changes in my belly and in how my clothes fit. There was a pair of pants that I bought before this diet, and I said to myself, 'If I lose 5 pounds in the next 3 weeks, I'll keep them, and if I can't lose the weight, I'll return them.' Well, I'm keeping those pants!"

She also found herself "wanting to run—even while on vacation!" And her digestive issues vanished, except on the few occasions she veered off the plan and had some fried foods. Having lost 6 pounds despite all of these dieting challenges, she is motivated to keep eating the 21-Day Tummy way, thanks to her new attitude.

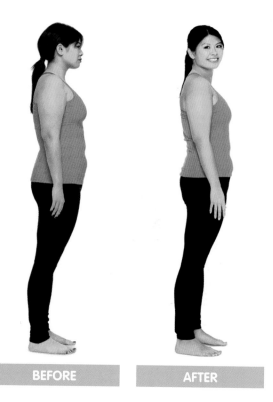

BEFORE   AFTER

Sabrina Ng

Age 31

Lost 6 POUNDS and 1¾ BELLY INCHES in 21 days!

Proudest accomplishments: Her clothes fit better; learning to love exercise; not letting travel derail her progress

Favorite meals: Curried Chicken Soup; Beef and Red Quinoa–Stuffed Eggplant

(continued from page 107)

stabilize your blood sugar and combat inflammation. Fresh is best, of course, but it's tough to find fresh coconut milk unless you live on a tropical island (if only!). Canned or boxed coconut milk can give you that island flavor in a jiffy; just avoid products that have added sugar. And because coconut milk is high in fat, we suggest that you go for low-fat or light versions and limit yourself to ¼ cup per serving. You may also want to look for varieties that are fortified with calcium.

Coconut water, by the way, is also great for you—what's marketed as coconut water is actually coconut juice, the liquid that's naturally sloshing around inside a young coconut. It contains lauric acid, along with other nutrients, and is lower in fat than coconut milk. Coconut oil, which is made from mature coconut meat, is rich in lauric acid, too, so, although it's high in saturated fats, it can make a good replacement occasionally for other cooking oils.

Belly Buddy #10: Ginger

Most of us are familiar with ginger as a remedy for nausea, but did you know it's also an anti-inflammatory and strengthens the muscle movements of your GI tract? In a double-blind study, 24 volunteers took either ginger tablets or a placebo. It took less time for the stomach to empty in those who took the ginger tablets, and muscle contractions in the abdomen (as measured by ultrasound) were more frequent.[18] All told, that's a great combination for creating a calm, happy system.

Ginger is very common in Asian food but can be used in a number of dishes—you can even grate it into salads, stir-fries, and sauces. It's a rootlike spice and keeps well even when fresh. Powdered ginger, ginger candy, and ginger tea also help, but fresh is better. Ginger is my go-to flavoring for my second-favorite Belly Soother Smoothie, the Creamsicle.

Belly Buddy #11: Turmeric

Turmeric, used in Indian curry, is a powerful antioxidant and may help fight infections and reduce inflammation. Research suggests that turmeric stimulates the gallbladder to produce more bile, which may improve digestion.[19]

Turmeric may also help relieve the symptoms of ulcerative colitis, according to research at the University of Maryland Medical Center. In one double-blind, placebo-controlled study, people whose colitis was in remission took either curcumin (the most active component of turmeric) or a placebo for 6 months. Those who took curcumin had a much lower relapse rate.[20]

Belly Buddy #12: Maple Syrup

Still have that sweet tooth? Kate recommends pure maple syrup, in moderation, because it has the lowest amount of fructose of its fellow sweeteners. After trying the Belly Bully Tests in Chapter 9, I realized that fructose is one of my Belly Bullies. The good-for-you honey that I'd been using to sweeten my tea for the last 20 years? Tossed it. Like table sugar, honey is high in excess fructose, which my body doesn't absorb very well. Agave nectar? Out. Agave is extremely high in excess fructose. Kate's exact words: "Off the charts!" Now, I drink my tea with just a sprinkle of cinnamon for flavor, and I use maple syrup to sweeten any of the smoothie concoctions that need it (few do).

***

Hungry yet? Now you understand how carb-dense foods, FODMAPs, and pro-inflammatory fats bully your belly with gas and bloating, heartburn and acid reflux, constipation, diarrhea, and IBS. You know how to find carb-light, low-FODMAP, high-fiber, and magnesium-rich Belly Buddies to help heal your tummy. It's time to put this information into action. Get ready for the best belly you've ever had: your 21-Day Tummy!

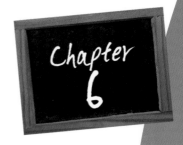

Chapter 6

The 21-Day Tummy Meal Plan

Here's the moment you've been waiting for. Time to dig into the 21-Day Tummy diet—the meal plan that helped me and all 11 of my fellow testers shrink our stomachs (by up to 4½ inches in one case!) and soothe our tummy troubles. At least two people were able to stop taking prescription medications for heartburn entirely, and GI symptoms disappeared completely for several testers. The rest of us noticed that the few times we had a little gas or a mild stomach cramp, we had eaten something that was not on the plan—proof that if you stick with it, this diet works!

21 Days to the Tummy You Always Wanted

Let's recap: In order to balance your gut microbiota and cool inflammation, the 21-Day Tummy diet radically restricts Belly Bullies such as refined carbs and grains and goes delightfully wild with increased consumption of Belly Buddies, including many colorful vegetables and fruits.

It means eating:

1. **More magnesium-rich foods.** Magnesium deficiency is linked to obesity and inflammation. The 21-Day Tummy diet loads up on spinach, brown rice, and pumpkin seeds, among other whole foods, to provide more of this vital mineral.

2. **More anti-inflammatory fats.** Pair the MUFAs that specifically target visceral belly fat with the omega-3s that combat inflammation and the many diseases associated with it. This protects you from heart disease, depression, type 2 diabetes, stroke, cancer, and, of course, gastrointestinal disorders and weight gain.

3. **Fewer carb-dense foods.** To minimize carb-dense foods, the 21-Day Tummy diet cuts out sugar, refined carbs, and most grains. Instead, it adds carb-light, natural foods like bananas, potatoes, and leafy green vegetables. Lean proteins and healthy fats are also carb-light.

4. **Fewer FODMAPs.** Clear your system of the rapidly fermentable carbs or sugars that can play an ugly role in your digestive system, causing gas, bloating, diarrhea, and constipation. Everything from the fructose in agave nectar to the lactose in milk can

be fast food for the bacteria in your gut, which is bad news for those of us with sensitive stomachs. The 21-Day Tummy diet minimizes FODMAPs, then guides you through a test to see which ones you can tolerate after 3 weeks.

By now I hope I've convinced you that Belly Buddies really do work miracles for your tummy. But you may be unsure of what to do with some of these foods. It's easy enough to nosh on berries and grapes, or to throw together a quick salad with cucumbers and carrots. But how do you cook quinoa? Since you can't have pancakes, what do you do with maple syrup? What pairs well with parsnips?

> The Belly Soother Smoothie is an endlessly versatile and refreshing power drink that helps replace some meals.

The 21-Day Tummy meal plan pulls the Belly Buddies together into three delicious and satisfying meals each day plus one scrumptious snack. Kate made sure each day is packed with a variety of Belly Buddies so you never get bored. At the same time, we worked hard to make good use of leftovers throughout the plan. I wanted to reduce the amount of cooking and ensure that no food goes to waste.

Kate has carefully constructed meals to balance nutrients. She's also worked in some probiotic foods to help balance gut flora and reduce gas and bloating. And she developed the Belly Soother Smoothie, an endlessly versatile and refreshing power drink that helps replace some meals. (I start every day with a different variation!)

The 21-Day Tummy diet consists of three phases:

PHASE 1: FLATTEN (Days 1–5)

In this stage of the plan, you'll pacify your sensitive system while shedding fat quickly. In order to jump-start your weight loss, this phase is lowest in calories, replacing one meal per day with the Belly Soother Smoothie. While we don't recommend restricting calories for too long, doing so at this stage helps you get results fast so you're motivated to stick with the diet. And don't worry—while this is a lower-calorie phase, it's hardly a starvation diet. You'll be enjoying hearty soups, big salads, and tender grilled chicken and pork with baked potato and veggies on the side. I find this phase the easiest to follow and the most cleansing, satisfying five days of any diet I've tried.

The Flatten phase is also designed to nourish and soothe your belly. It's very low in FODMAP foods and contains no grains (even the Belly Buddies oats, oat bran, quinoa, polenta, and buckwheat are not introduced until later). Here, we focus on the foods that are the absolute easiest to digest healthfully. Once we've cleaned out our digestive systems, we can slowly introduce foods that take a little more work, such as the grains on the Belly Buddy list. Listen up: While I promise you will immediately feel leaner and cleaner on this phase, this is not a "detox" diet of liquid meals or bland foods. This phase is about eating real food—and getting real results. Our testers lost an average of 5½ pounds after this phase!

ME AND MY "STUMBLE-UPON FOODS"

I first realized I ate stumble-upon foods one steaming hot August morning years ago. I was walking down a Manhattan street, and a nice young man stood outside a new deli holding a tray of muffin pieces for passersby. As I reached for a piece of iced blueberry scone that had probably been manhandled by a dozen sweaty commuter fingers, I thought, "What am I doing?!"

By stumble-upon foods, I mean candy on the work giveaway table, platters of bagels in a meeting, mints at restaurant checkouts, food in cups at grocery store tasting stations. Stumble-upon foods are foods you don't seek out, but eat anyway because they're there and they're free.

I was eyeing the same platter of cookies yesterday as a fellow tester, and it led to a good conversation about foods that pop up out of the blue and tempt us. "Funny how when I have a plan of what to eat (instead of just winging it), it's so much easier to pass up all the 'stumble-upon foods,'" I said.

PHASE 2: SOOTHE AND SHRINK (Days 6–15)

For the next 10 days, you'll maximize belly fat loss by boosting anti-inflammatory foods rich in magnesium and monounsaturated fatty acids. You'll continue to enjoy one Belly Soother Smoothie per day, but your other meals will be larger to keep your metabolism humming. Since meals are a little bigger, allow at least 2 to 3 hours between eating. This helps give your digestive system a break and allows your small intestine to be adequately cleaned out between meals.

In Phase 2, we introduce quinoa and oat bran, the most carb-light of grains. Oat bran and quinoa are also both rich in magnesium. They're paired with magnesium-rich fruits, veggies, nuts, and seeds, plus MUFA-rich oils and other foods, to create filling stir-fries and chicken dinners that will keep you fueled up and feeling good.

PHASE 3: BALANCE (Days 16–21)

In our final phase, you'll enjoy balanced meals that combine belly-friendly fiber, lean protein, and healthy fats to "lock and load your body" so you are never chasing hunger. Meals in this phase feature an ideal balance of 40 percent carbs, 30 percent protein, and 30 percent fat. Research indicates that that's the best mix to decrease inflammation and improve digestion so it's the combination we recommend you stick with for life.[1]

In Phase 3, we add in small portions of low-FODMAP grains, including oats, buckwheat, polenta, and brown rice, which boost your serotonin levels and improve your mood without derailing your weight loss or destabilizing your tummy. We'll stay largely carb-light, but now you're ready to reintroduce sweets to your diet, with a delicious dessert every other day.

Frequently Asked Questions

Our test team raised a lot of questions during the plan, and I bet you're wondering some of the same things. I've included the questions and answers below.

1. **Can I swap meals within the plan?**

   Yes, as long as they're similar. For instance, swap one soup that doesn't appeal to you for a soup that does. Also, while you can always have a meal from an earlier phase, don't sub in a meal from a later phase.

2. **Am I allowed to have any alcohol?**

   Ideally, no. Alcohol can irritate your digestive tract and draw water into your intestine, leading to diarrhea. Plus, alcohol contains empty calories. A few types of drinks can be especially troubling—rum and most dessert wines are high in fructose and beer contains gluten. If you really want a drink, red and white wines seem to be least problematic for most people's tummies, perhaps because they have a relatively low carb content.

3. **Can I have soda?**

   No. And that means no regular or diet soda. Contrary to popular belief, the carbonation isn't the problem; it's the sweeteners (both artificial and natural), which often contain FODMAPs or fake chemicals. Seltzer water is a good substitute. It will give you the fizz you're looking for without the sweeteners and calories.

4. **What's the deal with caffeine?**

   If you're prone to constipation, caffeine can give your sluggish intestine a little kick to get it moving. But if you tend to have diarrhea, you may want to steer clear of caffeine; it can be a troublemaker.

(continued on page 120)

YOUR TRAVELING TUMMY

Because traveling can be a hazard to your tummy (consider traveler's diarrhea and motion sickness), it's especially important to stick to healthy eating habits while you're away from home. Try these tips:

- Bring snacks with you. Some good choices include string cheese, small packets of nuts, celery and carrot sticks, oranges and bananas, maybe even some chia seeds or ground flaxseed for a fiber boost on the go!
- Pack a large garden salad with chicken or perhaps a Belly Soother Smoothie on travel days.
- Don't skip meals! At a minimum, be sure to have a piece of fruit and a handful of nuts if you're in a rush.
- Choose restaurants carefully (avoid all-you-can-eat buffets), scan menus before you head out, and opt for steamed, poached, broiled, baked, grilled, roasted, stir-fried, or lightly sautéed foods.
- Once at your destination, stop in at a local grocery store to stock up on easy breakfasts and snacks. Some items on your shopping list might include: instant oats, lactose-free milk, Greek yogurt, nuts, and fresh fruits and veggies.

When eating out, look for these options:

- Plain nonfat Greek yogurt, banana, and a handful of nuts (but no cashews or pistachios)
- Banana and peanut butter
- Hard-cooked or poached eggs on a bed of spinach with sliced almonds and chopped melon, berries (but no blackberries), or orange
- Egg white omelet with sautéed greens, a small amount of cheddar, and chopped melon, berries (but no blackberries), or orange
- Garden salad topped with grilled chicken or shrimp, dressed with vinegar and a dash of olive oil; ½ baked sweet potato or potato with skin (avoid heavy topping such as bacon bits, cheese and sour cream; a smear of butter or drizzle of olive oil is okay)
- Grilled fish with green beans or zucchini; a small garden salad with vinegar and a dash of olive oil
- Sushi (avoid mayo-based rolls like spicy tuna) and a garden or caprese salad with vinegar and a dash of olive oil
- Filet mignon; ½ baked sweet potato or potato with skin (avoid heavy topping such as bacon bits, cheese and sour cream; a smear of butter or drizzle of olive oil is okay); a small garden salad with vinegar and a dash of olive oil
- Asian-style vegetable stir-fry (no onions or garlic) with tofu, shrimp, or chicken and a handful of nuts; in Phase 3, a scoop of brown rice

(continued from page 118)

Also, beware of the FODMAPs that might lurk in your caffeinated beverage of choice. For me, both lactose and fructose can cause problems, so now I limit myself to just a splash of milk and a little cinnamon in my tea (no sugar). No more afternoon bloat!

Hot off the press: Instant coffee has FODMAPs so go for a brewed cup of Joe instead.

5. **What if I get hungry?**

Try drinking more water. Often, we think we're hungry when we're really just thirsty. Munching on fresh raw veggies also curbs hunger. Just be sure to pick veggies from the Belly Buddy list.

If you're really tall (over 6 feet) or extremely active (working out more than an hour a day), you may need a little more to keep you going. In that case, try adding another snack.

6. **Do I need to use lactose-free milk if I'm not lactose-intolerant?**

For this plan, it's best to stick with the lactose-free milk just in case you're sensitive to lactose and don't know it yet. You can add regular milk after the plan to see if you digest it well.

7. **Does the timing of meals matter?**

In order to push fiber and bacteria out, your small intestine initiates cleansing waves when you're in a fasting state. That only occurs about 2 hours or so after you eat, so it's best to leave 2 to 3 hours between each meal to give your intestines some time to fully clear out. You don't want your bacteria to linger in your small intestine as this increases your risk of small intestinal bacterial overgrowth.

Also, you want to space meals out throughout the

day so you never get too hungry (and then overeat) or too full (and then get indigestion). But don't stress about it if you can't eat exactly every 4 hours or if you wind up having breakfast and lunch back-to-back.

8. **My tummy's calmer on this diet, but I have to admit, I really miss my stuffed artichokes/watermelon/chili powder, etc. Will I be able to have it again?**

    I don't believe in forbidding any foods. But, as you've already figured out, a lot of your old favorites are probably responsible for your tummy troubles. After you finish the 21-day meal plan and have cleared your stomach of anything problematic, you can experiment with adding some of these foods back to see if they still bother you and if so, in what amounts. With spice mixes, the spices themselves are usually not the problem but the fact that they are blended with garlic and onion. Look for brands without these ingredients (see box on page 153 for suggestions).

9. **How do you introduce flavor without garlic or onions?**

    I know that garlic and onions are staples in most kitchens; they were in mine! Infusing olive oil with garlic or onion is a neat trick for getting the flavor you love without the FODMAPs. You can also use the green parts of scallions and chives; only the white parts contain FODMAPs.

> **TUMMY TWISTER OR TAMER? Hot Sauce**
>
> Tolerance to hot sauce is very individual. It's more problematic for those with heartburn. If you would like to try some, pick a brand without onion and garlic.

But these are hardly the only foods that can add flavor. Remember that many spices help you break down fat, so experiment! Ginger and turmeric are Belly Buddies so you'll see them featured in the meal plan. Smoked paprika and cumin can help round out the aroma of your dishes. Spice mixes like curry powder (which contains turmeric) and chili powder are also great options; just make sure you buy brands that are onion- and garlic-free.

10. **Every time I've tried dieting, I've ended up bingeing instead. Can you explain why?**

In short, we binge when there are other voids in our life. That's why forbidding foods rarely works. Lowered levels of the mood-boosting chemical serotonin in the brain may also contribute. Since, as we know, carb-rich foods help increase serotonin levels, cravings for those foods may be our body's way of increasing this brain chemical. That's why, on this diet, Kate made sure we kept enough carbs in to keep our serotonin levels up, so you won't be subject to those uncontrollable cravings.

11. **If something is gluten free, does that mean it's automatically low in FODMAPs?**

No. A gluten-free item is wheat free, barley free, and rye free. But other FODMAPs can sneak into the product, such as apple juice, chicory root extract (inulin), honey, agave syrup, or even garlic or onion.

12. **Can I dine out on this plan?**

Absolutely! While I encourage you to cook more so that you can better control what goes into your body, I don't want you to become a hermit. In fact, several of our testers did a lot of eating out. Rob McMahon and I both traveled for business, Jonathan Bigham survived a family trip to Disney World, and Sabrina Ng enjoyed an all-inclusive bachelorette party weekend in the Bahamas—all without ruining our diets or experiencing flare-ups of our digestive issues. See "Your Traveling Tummy" on page 119 for some tips.

The 21-Day Tummy Meal Plan

Your complete 21-day meal plan includes a mix of recipes and quick-fix meals. I suggest that you spend a little time each weekend reading through the upcoming week's menu and doing a little shopping and prepping.

Please note that the quick-fix meals in the plan all make individual portions. However, the recipes serve four (or sometimes more). We've done it this way so you can share the recipes with your family (if you usually cook for them) or you can freeze extra portions to use later. (In fact, you'll see that Kate has suggested doing this in a few instances.) To be sure you are eating single servings, note the portion amount given with each recipe.

SPECIAL NOTE ABOUT GLUTEN

If you have celiac disease, please look out for ingredients in the meal plan we've marked with an asterisk (*). These are foods that may contain gluten. The trace amounts found in these foods may be tolerated by people with nonceliac gluten sensitivity, but to be safe, look for gluten-free versions. See page 153 for recommended brands.

COMMON INGREDIENT SUBSTITUTIONS

If you are allergic to an ingredient called for in the meal plan, can't find it in the store, or simply hate it, here are some common substitutions you can make.

Lactose-free milk	Rice milk, light coconut milk†
Lactose-free cottage cheese	Farmer cheese (a low-lactose soft cheese), Greek yogurt (plain if using for dips)
Greens: arugula, kale, romaine, spinach, Swiss chard	Interchange as desired
Cabbage: green, red	Interchange as desired
Turnips	Parsnips, potatoes
Kiwi, star fruit	½ cup strawberries or blueberries
Papaya	Pineapple
Red quinoa	White or any other type of quinoa, brown rice
Chia seeds	Ground flaxseed or pumpkin seeds (pepitas)
Lean protein: fish, turkey tenderloin, chicken breast, pork tenderloin, lean beef	Interchange as desired

†Rice milk and coconut milk are not preferred because they have less protein.

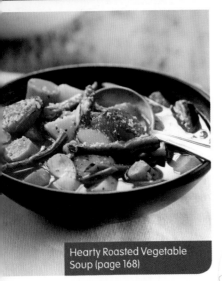

Grilled Chicken, Sweet Potato, and Kiwi Salad (page 191)

Hearty Roasted Vegetable Soup (page 168)

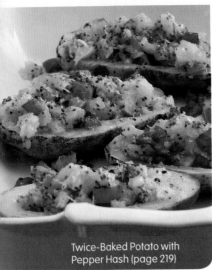

Twice-Baked Potato with Pepper Hash (page 219)

MAKE-AHEAD **MEALS**

If you start the diet on a Monday, it may help to do some cooking on the weekend. (In general, note that most cooked foods will keep in the refrigerator for 3 to 4 days and in the freezer for up to 3 months.) Here are some Sunday prep suggestions:

For Week 1   *Roasted garlic oil (211)*

- X • Roast, bake, or grill 7 ounces boneless, skinless chicken breast and refrigerate.

- X • Make **Mustard-y Dressing (page 208)**.

- • Make **Curried Chicken Soup (page 164)** or Caldo Verde **(page 166)** and refrigerate.

- X • Make **Grilled Chicken, Sweet Potato, and Kiwi Salad (page 191; pictured at top left)** and refrigerate but don't add kiwi until ready to serve.

- X • Make **Hearty Roasted Vegetable Soup (page 168; pictured at middle left)** and refrigerate or freeze.

- • Make **Twice-Baked Potato with Pepper Hash (page 219; pictured at bottom left)** and refrigerate (but do not freeze). *Fri Night*

- • Make **Beef and Red Quinoa-Stuffed Eggplant (page 185; pictured at top right)** and refrigerate (but do not freeze). *Sat Night*

For Week 2

- • Make **Mustard-y Dressing (page 208)** and **Asian Sesame Dressing (page 208)**.

- • Make **Cheesy Scrambled Egg "Quesadillas" (page 159; pictured at middle right)** and refrigerate or freeze.

- Make sauce for **Tuna Romesco (page 177)** and refrigerate.

- Make **Nutty Red Quinoa (page 220)** and refrigerate or freeze.

- Make **Pork Satay Salad (page 186; pictured at bottom right)** and refrigerate but don't add papaya until ready to serve.

- Make **Mini Quiches (page 160)** and refrigerate or freeze.

- Make **Creamy Chard and Spinach Soup (page 167)** and refrigerate or freeze.

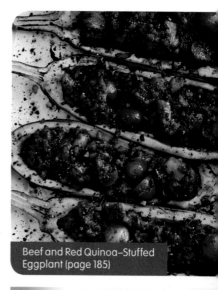

Beef and Red Quinoa–Stuffed Eggplant (page 185)

For Week 3

- Roast, bake, or grill 7 ounces boneless, skinless chicken breast and refrigerate.

- Cook 1 cup (dry) oat bran cereal per package directions; add cinnamon and ground ginger. Refrigerate to use in the **Creamy Oats and Yogurt Parfait (page 144)**.

- Cook ¼ cup (dry) brown rice and refrigerate to use in the **Steak Rice Bowl (page 144)**.

- Make **Mustard-y Dressing (page 208)** and **Asian Sesame Dressing (page 208)**.

- Make **Toasted Brown Rice and Pepper Pilaf (page 222)** and refrigerate (but do not freeze).

- Make **Toasted Almond Raspberry Muffins (page 162)** and freeze.

- Make **Kiwi-Glazed Turkey Meat Loaf (page 173)** and freeze.

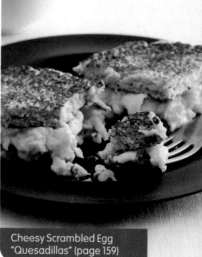

Cheesy Scrambled Egg "Quesadillas" (page 159)

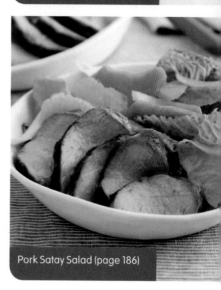

Pork Satay Salad (page 186)

Breakfast

Belly Soother Smoothie (page 156)

Lunch

Select either *Curried Chicken Soup (page 164)* or *Caldo Verde (page 166)*. Have 1 serving and save a serving for Day 3. Enjoy with ½ cup nonfat lactose-free milk and 10 red grapes.

or banana & pb

Snack

Curried Yogurt Dip: Combine ¼ cup nonfat plain Greek yogurt* with a dash of curry powder (ideally onion free, such as Spice Appeal) topped with 1 tablespoon pumpkin seeds. Dip and enjoy with 10 baby carrots.

Dinner

Balsamic Chicken: Roast, bake, or grill 7 ounces boneless, skinless chicken breast (or buy unseasoned cooked chicken, about 1 cup) and drizzle with balsamic vinegar. (Eat half and save the rest for tomorrow's lunch.) Serve with 2 cups sautéed or grilled zucchini brushed with 1 teaspoon olive oil, and ½ baked or grilled sweet potato. Before serving, top the potato with 1 teaspoon maple syrup, a dash of cinnamon, and 1 tablespoon chopped walnuts. Enjoy with a kiwi.

Breakfast

Belly Soother Smoothie (page 156)

Lunch

Go Go Greens! Kale and Chicken Salad: Toss 2 cups slivered kale or baby spinach with 1 tablespoon *Mustard-y Dressing (page 208)*. Top with the chicken left over from dinner on Day 1 (slice or shred it first) and a sprinkle of chia seeds.* Enjoy with ½ cup sliced strawberries.

Snack

Crunch and Go! 10 almonds, 1 mini cheese, and 10 baby carrots

Dinner

Lemony Salmon, Potato and Dill Bake (page 194) and 10 red grapes

Breakfast

Belly Soother Smoothie (page 156)

Lunch

Repeat a serving of soup from Day 1. Serve with 1 cup strawberries.

Snack

Fit 'n' Fruity Flax Parfait: Combine ½ cup nonfat plain Greek yogurt,* 1 teaspoon vanilla extract or vanilla paste, and ½ cup blueberries. Top with 1 tablespoon ground flaxseed.

Dinner

Mustard-Rubbed Pork Cutlet: Spread 2 teaspoons Dijon mustard* on top of a 4-ounce boneless center cut pork chop, sprinkle with a dash of sea salt and paprika, and roast in the oven with 1 medium red-skinned potato. When ready to serve, top the potato with 2 tablespoons nonfat plain Greek yogurt* and a sprinkle of chopped chives. Enjoy with 2 cups spinach, wilted in a skillet with 1 teaspoon reduced-sodium soy sauce* and 1 teaspoon sesame oil.

Breakfast

Belly Soother Smoothie (page 156)

Lunch

Grilled Chicken, Sweet Potato, and Kiwi Salad (page 191)

Snack

PB & B: Have 1 small banana with 2 teaspoons peanut butter, and enjoy with 1 cup nonfat lactose-free milk. Or, toss all the ingredients in the blender with ice for a cool, refreshing drink!

Dinner

Go Fish with Papaya Salsa: Mix ½ cup chopped papaya (you can substitute canned pineapple chunks if you can't find papaya) with 1 tablespoon chopped chives; ½ jalapeño chile pepper, chopped; ½ cup chopped red bell pepper; 1 tablespoon lime juice; 1 teaspoon olive oil; 2 tablespoons chopped cilantro; and salt and pepper to taste. Serve on top of 6 ounces baked or grilled halibut, cod, or tilapia. Enjoy with **Swiss Chard Sauté:** Sauté 2 cups Swiss chard in 2 teaspoons garlic-infused oil (you can either purchase or make the Roasted Garlic Oil on page 211), ½ teaspoon cumin, and 2 teaspoons minced ginger (you can sub ¼ teaspoon dry ginger); cook until just wilted.

Breakfast

Belly Soother Smoothie (page 156)

Lunch

Hearty Roasted Vegetable Soup (page 168): Save a serving for
   Day 7 dinner.

Snack

Mini Caprese Salad: Combine 10 grape tomatoes,
   1 mozzarella mini cheese (cut into 5 small pieces), and
   2 chopped basil leaves. Drizzle with balsamic vinegar.

Dinner

Tuna and Caesar Salad: Toss 2 cups shredded romaine
   with 1 tablespoon *Mustard-y Dressing (page 208)* and
   1 tablespoon shredded Parmesan cheese; top with one
   5-ounce can solid white tuna, packed in water (drained and
   rinsed). Season the tuna with fresh lemon juice. Enjoy with
   Twice-Baked Potato with Pepper Hash (page 219) and 1 cup
   cantaloupe chunks.

Breakfast

Belly Soother Smoothie (page 156)

Lunch

Go Greens! Roast, bake, or grill 4 ounces boneless, skinless chicken breast (or buy unseasoned cooked chicken, about ½ cup). Toss 2 cups salad greens of choice, 1 sliced celery stalk, and 1 tablespoon fresh basil with 1 tablespoon *Asian Sesame Dressing (page 208)*. Top with the chicken (slice or shred first). Enjoy with 1 cup blueberries and 1 cup nonfat lactose-free milk.

Snack

Crunch and Go! 10 almonds, 1 mini cheese, and 10 baby carrots

Dinner

Beef and Red Quinoa–Stuffed Eggplant (page 185). Save a serving of this dish for dinner on Day 8. Serve with 2 cups bok choy sautéed with 1 teaspoon reduced-sodium soy sauce* and 1 teaspoon sesame oil. Enjoy with 1 cup chopped cantaloupe.

Breakfast

Belly Soother Smoothie (page 156)

Lunch

Savory Shrimp and Greens: Toss 2 cups arugula, kale, spinach, or romaine with 2 teaspoons *Mustard-y Dressing (page 208)*, 1 tablespoon grated Parmesan cheese, and 2 tablespoons chopped pecans, walnuts, almonds, or pine nuts. Top with 6 large shrimp, roasted or boiled (can be served warm or chilled). Enjoy with an orange and 1 cup nonfat lactose-free milk.

Snack

PB & C: Spread 1 tablespoon peanut butter on 1 medium celery stalk. Enjoy with ½ cup nonfat lactose-free milk (or 1 mini cheese) and 10 red grapes.

Dinner

Hearty Roasted Vegetable Soup (left over from Day 5). Enjoy with a banana and 10 almonds.

Breakfast

Cheesy Scrambled Egg "Quesadillas" (page 159) and a banana

Lunch

Belly Soother Smoothie (page 156) and 10 almonds

Snack

Dilly Cheese Dip: Mix ½ cup low-fat lactose-free cottage cheese with a sprinkle of dill and a dash of turmeric. Enjoy as a dip with 10 baby carrots and 20 peanuts.

Dinner

Beef and Red Quinoa–Stuffed Eggplant (left over from Day 6). Enjoy with 1 cup chopped cantaloupe, 1 cup romaine lettuce with 2 teaspoons *Mustard-y Dressing (page 208),* and 1 cup nonfat lactose-free milk.

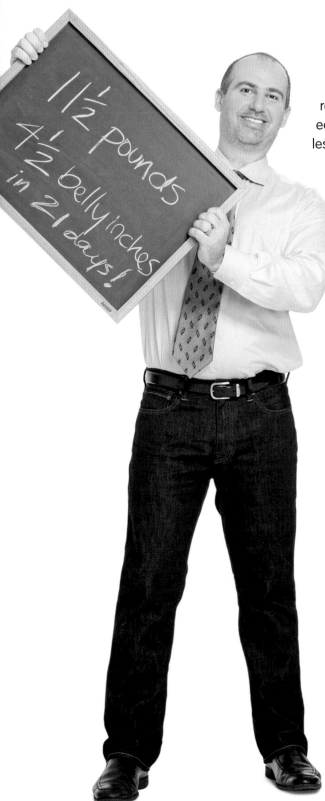

Gregg Roth is now feeling much more athletic. With his 21-Day Tummy, he reports, "I am able to play basketball a lot easier. I feel lighter on my feet and have less pain in my joints. I have more energy, and I feel less sluggish. I'm sleeping much better, too." It's amazing what a difference dropping 11½ pounds can make!

Plus, he says, "This diet was much better for digestion than other diets I've done. My digestion definitely improved. I was in Florida for 5 days and went off the plan, and I could tell there was a huge

More Athletic and Happier in 3 Weeks!

difference in my digestive system. Let's just say it was a gas thing. That went away as soon as I went back on the plan."

After that experience, Gregg learned how to stick with the plan even while traveling. He learned he could always stick with a few basic meals and how to substitute belly-friendly ingredients when a restaurant didn't have a specific dish. Now he's in the habit of making healthy choices everywhere. "When I'm out at a restaurant, instead of picking the cheeseburger with fries, I'm getting vegetable main dishes and lean proteins and things like that."

Not a cook himself, Gregg was nervous about trying new foods and recipes. Luckily, his wife was willing to help him with a lot of the cooking, but it was still a challenge. It's one he's glad he took up, though. "My health is much better than 3 weeks ago," he reports. "I'm just happier all around, and I want to hold on to that. You have to be prepared to put in some time, but the results are worth it."

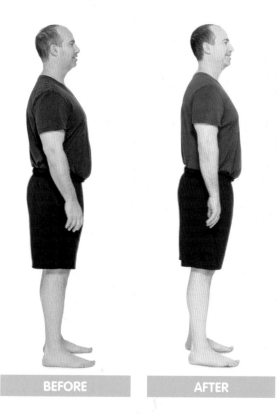

BEFORE AFTER

Gregg Roth

Age 47

Lost 11½ POUNDS and 4½ BELLY INCHES in 21 days!

Proudest accomplishments: Trimmed his tummy more than any other tester; learned to make healthy choices when eating out.

Favorite meals: Mustard-Rubbed Pork Chops; Belly Soother Smoothie

Breakfast

Belly Soother Smoothie (page 156)

Lunch

Sweet 'n' Sour Salad: Roast, bake, or grill 7 ounces boneless, skinless chicken breast (or buy unseasoned cooked chicken, about 1 cup). Toss 2 cups thinly sliced romaine lettuce with 2 chopped scallions (green part only), ¼ cup sliced water chestnuts, ½ cup mandarin oranges (drained of juice), and 2 teaspoons *Asian Sesame Dressing (page 208)*. Top with half the chicken (slice or shred it first) and a sprinkle of chia seeds.* (Save the rest of the chicken for tomorrow's lunch.)

Snack

PB & C: Spread 2 teaspoons peanut butter inside 1 medium celery stalk. Enjoy with 1 cup nonfat lactose-free milk.

Dinner

Tuna Romesco (page 177); medium baked or grilled (or even microwaved) red-skinned or Yukon Gold potato drizzled with 1 teaspoon garlic-infused oil (you can either purchase or make the Roasted Garlic Oil on page 211); 2 cups arugula tossed with 1 tablespoon fresh lemon juice, 1 teaspoon olive oil, and a dash of salt/pepper to taste. Enjoy with 1 cup mixed berries (raspberries, strawberries, and/or blueberries).

Breakfast

Belly Soother Smoothie (page 156)

Lunch

Nutty Red Quinoa (page 220) topped with the chicken left over from lunch on Day 9. Enjoy with an orange.

Snack

Carrot Cake Parfait: Mix ½ cup nonfat vanilla Greek yogurt,* a dash of cinnamon, and ¼ cup grated carrots and top with 1 tablespoon chopped walnuts.

Dinner

Pork Satay Salad (page 186), 1 cup nonfat lactose-free milk, and 1 cup mixed berries topped with 1 tablespoon chopped nuts

Breakfast

Belly Soother Smoothie (page 156)

Lunch

Crunchy Chopped Salad (page 202) with 6 large shrimp, roasted or boiled (can be served warm or chilled). Enjoy with 1 banana spread with 2 teaspoons peanut butter.

Snack

Crunch and Go! 10 almonds, 1 mini cheese, and 10 baby carrots

Dinner

Pork Stir Fry: 4 ounces boneless center cut pork chop, sliced in strips and sautéed in 2 teaspoons peanut oil (or substitute garlic-infused oil; you can either purchase or make the Roasted Garlic Oil on page 211) for 2 minutes; then add 2 cups bean sprouts, 2 thinly sliced carrots, and 1 cup chopped red and yellow bell peppers and cook; sprinkle with 1 tablespoon sliced almonds. Enjoy with a kiwi and ½ cup nonfat lactose-free milk.

Breakfast

Mini Quiches (page 160) (make the full recipe and freeze 1
   serving for breakfast on Day 19) and a medium banana

Lunch

Belly Soother Smoothie (page 156)

Snack

Mini Caprese Salad: Combine 10 grape tomatoes,
   1 mozzarella mini cheese (cut into 5 small pieces), and
   2 chopped basil leaves. Drizzle with balsamic vinegar.

Dinner

Roasted Chicken: Roast 7 ounces boneless, skinless chicken
   breast (or buy unseasoned cooked chicken, about 1 cup).
   Eat half with *Grape and Walnut Waldorf Salad (page 204)*,
   Nutty Red Quinoa (page 220), and 1 cup nonfat lactose-free
   milk. (Save the rest of the chicken for lunch on Day 14.)

Breakfast

Belly Soother Smoothie (page 156)

Lunch

Creamy Chard and Spinach Soup (page 167): Save a serving
for lunch on Day 15. Enjoy with ½ cup lactose-free cottage
cheese, cucumber spears, red bell pepper slices, and an
orange.

Snack

Crunch and Go! 10 almonds, 1 mini cheese, and 10 baby
carrots

Dinner

Salmon Steak Salad: 1 baked or grilled 5-ounce salmon
fillet and salad made with 2 cups chopped romaine lettuce,
10 grape or cherry tomatoes, 5 green olives, 5 or 6 cucumber
slices (from ½ cucumber; save the rest for your snack on
Day 15), and 2 teaspoons *Mustard-y Dressing (page 208)*.
Enjoy with a banana.

Breakfast

Belly Soother Smoothie (page 156)

Lunch

Sweet 'n' Sour Salad: Toss 2 cups thinly sliced romaine lettuce with 2 chopped scallions (green part only), ¼ cup sliced water chestnuts, ½ cup mandarin oranges (drained of juice), and 2 teaspoons *Asian Sesame Dressing (page 208).* Top with a sprinkle of chia seeds, 1 tablespoon chopped nuts (any kind except cashews or pistachios), and the chicken left over from Day 12 (slice or shred it first).

Snack

PB & B: Spread 2 teaspoons peanut butter on a banana. Enjoy with 1 cup nonfat lactose-free milk.

Dinner

Curry-Rubbed Chicken with Fresh Pineapple Chutney (page 174): Serve with 2 cups arugula drizzled with 2 teaspoons *Mustard-y Dressing (page 208)* and topped with 2 tablespoons shredded Parmesan cheese and 1 tablespoon nuts (any kind except cashews or pistachios). Enjoy with an orange.

Breakfast

Belly Soother Smoothie (page 156)

Lunch

Creamy Chard and Spinach Soup (left over from Day 13). Serve with a banana and 10 almonds.

Snack

Spicy Dip: Mix 2 tablespoons nonfat plain Greek yogurt* with a dash of turmeric and cumin, 1 teaspoon chia seeds,* and sea salt. Enjoy with red bell pepper strips (from ½ pepper; save the rest for dinner) and cucumber spears (left over from Day 13).

Dinner

Antipasto Platter: Slice 1 eggplant, 2 small zucchini, ½ red bell pepper, and 1 medium red-skinned potato. Brush the vegetables with 2 teaspoons garlic-infused oil (you can either purchase or make the Roasted Garlic Oil on page 211) and a dash of sea salt. Grill or roast until fork-tender. (Save 1 zucchini for tomorrow's dinner.) At the same time, grill or roast 7 ounces boneless, skinless chicken breast (or buy unseasoned cooked chicken, about 1 cup). Place cooked veggies on a plate with 10 olives and half of the chicken (save the rest of the chicken for tomorrow's lunch). Top with chopped basil and 2 teaspoons *Mustard-y Dressing (page 208)*. Enjoy with an orange.

Breakfast

Spinach Scramble: Toss 1 cup baby spinach in a nonstick skillet with 2 teaspoons olive oil until spinach wilts (drain any extra liquid). Add ½ cup egg whites, ½ teaspoon Italian seasoning, and 2 tablespoons shredded reduced-fat cheddar cheese and heat until the eggs are cooked through. Enjoy with 1 banana and 1 cup nonfat lactose-free milk.

Lunch

Tomato Lime Quinoa Salad (page 205) (make the full recipe and save 1 serving for Day 19) topped with the chicken left over from dinner on Day 15 (slice or shred it first) and 1 tablespoon pumpkin seeds. Enjoy with 1½ cups cantaloupe chunks.

Snack

Orange and 10 almonds

Dinner

Tomato-Ginger Flank Steak (page 171) and *Toasted Brown Rice and Pepper Pilaf (page 222)*. Enjoy with 1 small roasted zucchini (left over from dinner on Day 15). (Save ½ cup sliced flank steak for tomorrow's lunch.)

Dessert

Chocolate Covered Strawberries (makes 2 servings): Place 1 tablespoon semisweet chocolate chips in a microwave-safe dish and melt in the microwave on regular power for 50 seconds, stirring halfway through. Dip 2 large strawberries halfway in chocolate and roll in 1 tablespoon finely chopped walnuts. Place on wax paper and chill in the refrigerator for 30 minutes or eat right away!

Breakfast

Creamy Oats and Yogurt Parfait: Cook ½ cup (dry) oat bran cereal* per package directions; add a dash of cinnamon and ground ginger and ½ cup chopped strawberries. Enjoy with 6 ounces nonfat plain Greek yogurt* mixed with 1 teaspoon vanilla, 1 tablespoon ground flaxseed, and 1 tablespoon chopped nuts (any kind except cashews or pistachios).

Lunch

Steak Rice Bowl: Place ⅓ cup cooked brown rice in the bottom of a salad bowl. Top with 2 cups spinach, the flank steak left over from dinner on Day 16, 5 baby carrots, 1 tablespoon chopped scallion (green part only), ½ cup mandarin oranges (drained of juice), and 1 tablespoon sliced almonds. Drizzle with 1 tablespoon *Asian Sesame Dressing (page 208)*.

Snack

Carrot Cake Parfait: Mix ½ cup nonfat vanilla Greek yogurt,* a dash of cinnamon, and ¼ cup grated carrots and top with 1 tablespoon chopped walnuts.

Dinner

Mustard Rubbed Pork Cutlet: Spread 2 teaspoons Dijon mustard* on top of a 4-ounce center cut boneless pork chop, sprinkle with a dash of sea salt and paprika, and roast in the oven with 1 medium red-skinned potato. When ready to serve, top the potato with 2 tablespoons nonfat plain Greek yogurt* and a sprinkle of chopped chives. Serve with 2 cups kale, Swiss chard, or spinach wilted in a skillet with 1 teaspoon reduced-sodium soy sauce* and 1 teaspoon sesame oil. Enjoy with 1 cup strawberries.

Breakfast

Toasted Almond Raspberry Muffins (page 162): Bake and
freeze in advance for quick heating and serving. Enjoy with
6 ounces nonfat plain Greek yogurt. Add a dash of vanilla
extract or vanilla paste and 1 teaspoon maple syrup to
sweeten it up!

Lunch

Go Greens! 2 cups greens (spinach, kale, arugula) topped
with 4 slices turkey deli meat* and 2 teaspoons *Asian
Sesame Dressing (page 208)* and 2 tablespoons pumpkin
seeds. Enjoy with 10 brown rice crackers* and 20 red
grapes.

Snack

Crunch and Go! 10 almonds, 1 mini cheese, and 10 baby
carrots

Dinner

Go Fish! 4 ounces broiled cod, haddock, or tilapia.
Serve with 2 cups steamed green beans or 2 cups salad
greens such as kale, spinach, or romaine lettuce drizzled
with 2 teaspoons *Mustard-y Dressing (page 208)* and
1 tablespoon sliced almonds. Enjoy with 1 cup blueberries.

Dessert

Peanut Butter–Banana Freeze (page 226)

Lauren Weiss

As a single girl in the city, Lauren was happy to have an active social life . . . but not so happy with how active her tummy was in response! With a "really easily upset stomach," Lauren regularly suffered from bloating, cramps, nausea, diarrhea, and "really bad heartburn." Still, she almost dropped out of the program before she even started because the cooking and shopping seemed too overwhelming. But she needed to make a real change in her lifestyle. And so she did! After 21 days, her symptoms had all faded, plus she had made a good start on weight loss, dropping 5 pounds and 2 inches from her waist.

Q: How was the 21-Day Tummy diet different from other diets you've tried?

A: My last diet was just counting calories and exercising. This diet helped me change my eating and taught me how to think about it, instead of just moderating food.

Q: What's changed since you started the diet?

A: The biggest change for me has been eating a healthy breakfast. The smoothies started me off the right way each morning, and I wasn't hungry quickly after them. And they were easy, which I need.

Q: What did you think about the recipes?

A: At first the recipes were kind of daunting because I don't normally use all those different spices. But once I tried them, I noticed that the food tasted a lot better than the processed food I was used to—and without adding a bunch of calories. There's lots of really easy meals and sides I can make quickly after work, or make in a big batch and have for lunch all week.

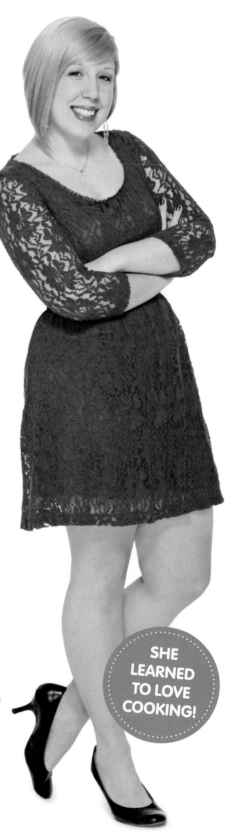

SHE LEARNED TO LOVE COOKING!

Breakfast

Mini Quiches (page 160) (left over from Day 12; to reheat, wrap in foil and reheat in the oven at 300 degrees Fahrenheit for about 10 minutes, or thaw overnight in the fridge and serve chilled or at room temperature). Enjoy with ¼ cup lactose-free cottage cheese and 1 cup mixed berries.

Lunch

Roast, bake, or grill 7 ounces boneless, skinless chicken breast (or buy unseasoned cooked chicken, about 1 cup). Top *Tomato Lime Quinoa Salad (page 205)* with half of the chicken (slice or shred it first). (Save the rest of the chicken for tomorrow's lunch.) Enjoy with a banana and 10 peanuts.

Snack

Fruit 'n' Nut Parfait: Combine ½ cup nonfat plain Greek yogurt, 1 teaspoon vanilla extract, and ½ cup blueberries. Top with 2 teaspoons ground flaxseed or 2 teaspoons sliced almonds.

Dinner

Kiwi-Glazed Turkey Meat Loaf (page 173) served with *Sesame Pasta (page 221)* and 2 cups bok choy sautéed and drizzled with 1 teaspoon sesame oil or garlic-infused oil (you can either purchase or make the Roasted Garlic Oil on page 211).

Breakfast

Creamy Oats and Yogurt Parfait: Cook ½ cup (dry) oat bran cereal* per package directions; add a dash of cinnamon and ground ginger and ½ cup chopped strawberries. Enjoy with 6 ounces nonfat plain Greek yogurt* mixed with 1 teaspoon vanilla, 1 tablespoon ground flaxseed, and 1 tablespoon chopped nuts (any kind except cashews or pistachios).

Lunch

Chicken and Caesar: Toss 2 cups shredded romaine with 2 teaspoons *Mustard-y Dressing (page 208)* and top with the chicken left over from lunch on Day 19. Enjoy with an orange and 10 brown rice crackers.*

Snack

Spicy Dip: Mix ¼ cup nonfat plain Greek yogurt* with a dash of turmeric, cumin, and sea salt, and enjoy with red bell pepper strips (from ½ red pepper) and cucumber spears (from ½ cucumber).

Dinner

Cheesy Tostada Pizzas: Sauté 4 ounces ground chicken with chili powder, cumin, and chopped cilantro. Top 2 corn tostada shells with the chicken, ½ cup chopped tomatoes, 2 tablespoons reduced-fat cheddar cheese,* and ⅓ cup *Easy Belly-Friendly Salsa (page 223)*. Enjoy with ¾ cup steamed sliced carrots and ½ cup diced pineapple.

Dessert

Plan ahead! Banana "Ice cream": Freeze ⅓ cup light coconut milk in an ice cube tray; cut 1 small banana into chunks and freeze. Combine these with 1 teaspoon vanilla extract and ¼ cup water in a blender until creamy.

Breakfast

Huevos Rancheros: Heat 2 corn tortillas in a skillet, then top with 2 poached or scrambled eggs, ⅓ cup shredded reduced-fat cheddar cheese, and ⅓ cup *Easy Belly-Friendly Salsa (page 223);* season with a dash of paprika and cumin, if desired. Enjoy with an orange.

Lunch

Mediterranean Couscous: Toss together ½ cup cooked brown rice couscous, 2 chopped scallions (green part only), 10 cherry tomatoes, 1 tablespoon feta cheese, and 2 teaspoons *Mustard-y Dressing (page 208).* Top with one 5-ounce can solid white tuna, packed in water (drained and rinsed). Enjoy with 10 red grapes.

Snack

Crunch and Go! 10 almonds, 1 mini cheese, and 10 baby carrots

Dinner

Mama Mia Burger: Mix 4 ounces ground chicken, 1 egg white, 1 tablespoon chopped chives, ¼ cup chopped red bell pepper, and a dash of Italian seasoning. Form a burger patty and grill. Enjoy with **Sweet Potato Fries:** Cut a small (5½-inch-long) sweet potato into steak fry shapes, coat evenly with 2 teaspoons olive oil and a dash of sea salt and paprika, and bake at 350°F for 30–40 minutes, turning occasionally. Serve with 2 cups steamed green beans (season with fresh lemon juice and dill, if desired).

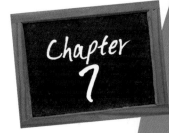
Chapter
7

Recipes That Shrink, Soothe, and Satisfy

When I look back on my childhood, dinnertime with my family looms large. Now that I have my own family, food continues to be an important bonding activity. I love to teach my daughters about healthy foods, to see their tastes change as they grow and try new foods. The time we spend together at the table is priceless. That's where we learn about each other's days, share stories, and plan for the future. And it's where we enjoy healthy (usually), yummy (always!) food that's the foundation of a calm and happy belly.

I hope these meals inspire some of *your* family's fondest memories and most meaningful conversations.

Making Meals That Shrink, Soothe, and Satisfy

The only way you're going to commit to eating well is if you like every bite, so I enlisted two of the best recipe developers in the business, Kate Slate and Sandra Gluck, to help me create recipes that will delight both your taste buds and your tummy. A happy surprise? Easy-to-digest does not mean bland. Sure, there are a few mild foods, like bananas, that happen to be great for your belly. But there are also some, like saltines, that turn out to be carb-dense and full of FODMAPs. Conversely, while hot sauce, garlic, and onions can irritate your digestive tract, the flavorful fresh ingredients of the 21-Day Tummy plan—including Belly Buddy spices like ginger and turmeric—help soothe the inflammation and microbial imbalance that trouble your tummy.

If you're in a rut, making the same five or 10 meals over and over, these recipes will add some pizzazz. It's so fun to try new foods and to try other foods for the first time in years. It always surprises me how the taste buds change. I've long thought I had an aversion to fish, which is why I'm stunned that one of my favorite 21-Day Tummy recipes is a fish dinner: the Lemony Salmon, Potato, and Dill Bake. Now I think of fish as a blank canvas, and what I serve on it or over it is the vibrant color. I like how light and healthy (yet satisfied) I feel after a dinner of fish with a side of greens. Talk about a life change! I even found myself trying a four-spice salmon recipe the other night. My husband was shocked by my choice, but not by how delicious it was.

I also made sure that the recipes in the 21-Day Tummy diet are quick and easy to make. You'll rarely find yourself in the kitchen for more than half an hour, and often you can be in and out in just 10 minutes.

> A happy surprise? Easy-to-digest does not mean bland.

In this chapter, you'll find all your favorite recipes from the 21-day plan plus some additional recipes that you can use to substitute for them if you choose. All of the recipes are carb-light (even the muffins only weigh in at about 30 grams of carbs per 100 grams) and chock-full of Belly Buddies, as you'll see from our call outs.

The recipes are organized by the type of dish, so you will find easy-to-prepare breakfasts, hearty soups, mouthwatering main courses, filling one-dish mains, sensational salads, simple sides, and of course, delectable desserts. For the most part, you can substitute within each category as long as you're in the appropriate phase. Note that you can always eat recipes from an earlier phase—in other words, in Phase 2, you can have any recipes from Phase 1 or 2; in Phase 3, you can have any of the recipes in this book.

RECOMMENDED BRANDS

Many spices and sauces, among other foods, may contain trace amounts of gluten. While most people with gluten intolerance can consume these without symptoms, for those with celiac disease these traces of gluten can be toxic! To be safe, we suggest that you look for brands known to be gluten free. Here are a few suggestions of gluten-free products to look for. Except where noted, these brands are also free of garlic and onions.

- Chobani nonfat plain Greek yogurt
- Fage nonfat plain Greek yogurt
- Laughing Cow Light Creamy Swiss spreadable cheese
- ReNew Life Ultimate ChiaLife
- Bob's Red Mill Gluten Free Oat Bran
- McCormick Chili Powder (contains onion)
- McCormick Chipotle Chile Pepper
- Spice Appeal Chili Powder
- Spice Appeal Curry Powder
- Pacific Organic Free Range Low Sodium Chicken Broth (contains onion)
- Lea & Perrins Worcestershire Sauce (contains onion)
- San-J Tamari Gluten-Free Soy Sauce
- Maille mustard
- Hunt's plain canned tomatoes
- Muir Glen fire-roasted canned tomatoes

Finally, if you're looking for lactose-free yogurt, try Green Valley Organics.

Many of the recipes are complete meals. In some cases, though, you'll want to add a little something to round out your meal. We've given you some appropriate suggestions, but some general guidelines may help:

- To breakfasts, add a Belly Buddy fruit (unless the recipe already includes a fruit).

- To main courses, add a simple salad or a side dish of leafy green vegetables.

- To the salads and sides, add 3 ounces of broiled, baked, grilled, or roasted lean beef, pork, or chicken (4 ounces raw) or 6 ounces of broiled, baked, grilled, or roasted fish or shrimp (fish and shrimp do not reduce in weight significantly during cooking, so you can start with 6 ounces raw).

And of course, you can always adapt the recipes themselves to suit your tastes or to make good use of produce or other ingredients you have in the house. Remember that you can always substitute ingredients as long as they are similar (protein for protein, fruit for fruit, etc.)—review the chart on page 123 for common swaps. Just steer clear of Belly Bullies listed in Chapter 4 while you experiment.

Keep in mind that the recipes here mostly make 4 servings; you will want to eat just 1 serving at each meal. If you live alone or your family refuses to eat your "diet food" (though after they see, smell, and taste the deliciousness coming from the kitchen, they may change their minds!), you can either cut the recipes accordingly or prepare them as written and save the other portions for meals later in the week (as we suggested in the 21-Day Tummy meal plan). We've given you tips for how to store extras, as well as suggestions for how to jazz up leftovers.

Breakfasts

Belly Soother Smoothie

full of BELLY BUDDIES to get you GOING!

← Creamsicle: Vanilla and Orange Collide!

Belly Soother Smoothie

Hands-On Time: 5 minutes | **Total Time:** 5 minutes | **Makes:** 1 smoothie

A refreshing and satisfying way to start your day, this smoothie is a key component of the 21-Day Tummy diet. Build on the base of creamy protein-rich Greek yogurt and coconut milk, both Belly Buddies, and add in different combinations of fruits that shrink and soothe your stomach, magnesium and fiber boosters that calm inflammation, and MUFAs that keep both your tummy and your taste buds happy!

Master Recipe:

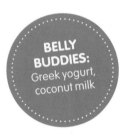

BELLY BUDDIES: Greek yogurt, coconut milk

6 ounces nonfat plain Greek yogurt

2 tablespoons light coconut milk

1–2 tablespoons water (frozen fruit requires more water than fresh)

1 teaspoon pure maple syrup (optional, for an extra hint of sweet)

4–6 ice cubes, or more, to create desired thickness; if using frozen fruits, omit ice

Add one of each from the following groups:

Fruit:

1 banana

1 cup strawberries

1 orange

2 kiwis

¾ cup cup blueberries

¾ cup raspberries

20 red grapes

½ cup cubed papaya

½ cup pineapple chunks

Magnesium and fiber booster:

1 tablespoon chia, flax, or pumpkin seeds

MUFAs

1 teaspoon peanut butter

1 teaspoon almond butter

Flavoring (choose one or more, if desired):

1 teaspoon unsweetened cocoa

½ teaspoon vanilla extract

¼ teaspoon ground cinnamon

1 teaspoon ground ginger, or 1 teaspoon grated or minced fresh ginger

A typical shake: Per serving: 281 calories • 20g protein • 8.5g fat (2g saturated) • 9g fiber • 35g carbohydrate • 79mg sodium • 59mg magnesium

If you are lactose intolerant: Reduce the yogurt to 4 ounces and up the coconut milk to 4 tablespoons. Or substitute lactose-free yogurt.

If you have gluten issues: Choose gluten-free brands of Greek yogurt and chia seeds.

Combine all of the ingredients in a blender and blend until frothy. Enjoy immediately.

Here are a few of my favorite flavor combinations. I hope they inspire you!

Creamsicle: Vanilla and orange collide

- 6 ounces nonfat plain Greek yogurt
- 2 tablespoons light coconut milk
- 1 orange, peeled and removed from membranes
- 1 tablespoon pumpkin seeds
- 1 teaspoon peanut butter
- 1 teaspoon fresh ginger, or ⅛ teaspoon ground ginger
- ½ teaspoon vanilla extract
- 6 ice cubes, or more to desired thickness

Chunky Chocolate: Hints of banana, peanut butter, and chocolate

- 6 ounces nonfat plain Greek yogurt
- 1 banana (peel and freeze the night before, or use at room temperature and add ice)
- 2 tablespoons light coconut milk
- 1 teaspoon maple syrup
- 1 tablespoon pumpkin seeds
- 1 teaspoon peanut butter
- 1 teaspoon unsweetened cocoa

Berry Good: Sweet and tangy!

- 6 ounces nonfat plain Greek yogurt
- ½ cup fresh or frozen blueberries
- ½ cup fresh or frozen strawberries
- 2 tablespoons light coconut milk
- 1 teaspoon maple syrup
- 1–2 tablespoons water
- 1 tablespoon chia seeds
- 1 teaspoon almond butter
- 1 teaspoon unsweetened cocoa

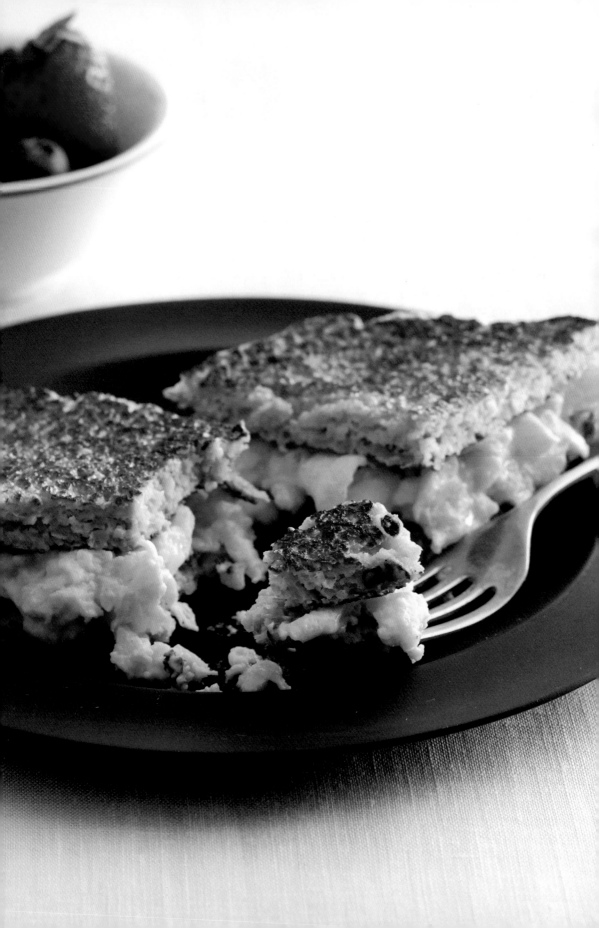

Cheesy Scrambled Egg "Quesadillas"

Hands-On Time: 20 minutes | **Total Time:** 20 minutes |
Makes: 4 (½ quesadilla) servings

This lean, protein-rich breakfast will leave you satisfied so you won't be tempted to eat for hours. You'll make your own quick and easy wrap for these quesadillas from carb-light oat bran. This recipe can be doubled or tripled, so whip up a batch of the oat wraps and freeze them in stacks (with layers of waxed paper in between) for super-quick breakfasts later. When you're ready to make the quesadillas, peel off the paper and reheat the wraps you need in the microwave or toaster oven for about a minute. Not in the mood for eggs? Top the wraps with your favorite berries and enjoy them as "pancakes."

3 large egg whites, or ½ cup liquid egg whites

½ cup nonfat plain Greek yogurt

½ cup oat bran

½ teaspoon salt

4 tablespoons water

Olive oil spray

4 large eggs

2 wedges (¾ ounce each) light spreadable cheese

BELLY BUDDIES:
Eggs, Greek yogurt, oat bran

1. In a large bowl, whisk together the egg whites, yogurt, oat bran, salt, and 2 tablespoons of the water until well combined.

2. Coat a large nonstick skillet with cooking spray. Spoon ⅓ cup of the mixture into the pan and, with a silicone spatula, spread it out to a 5-inch wrap. Cook for 15 seconds, or until golden brown on the underside and bubbles appear on the top. Flip the wrap over and cook for 15 seconds, or until the underside is done. Repeat with the remaining batter to make 4 wraps.

3. Off the heat, coat the same skillet with cooking spray. In a small bowl, whisk together the whole eggs and the remaining 2 tablespoons water. Heat the pan over low heat, add the eggs and cheese, and cook, stirring constantly, for 4 minutes, or until the eggs are just set.

4. Divide the eggs between 2 of the wraps, top with the remaining wraps, cut in half, and serve.

Per serving: 153 calories • 15g protein • 7.5g fat (2.5g saturated) • 2g fiber • 10g carbohydrate • 544mg sodium • 36mg magnesium

If you have gluten issues: Choose gluten-free brands of Greek yogurt, oat bran, and light spreadable cheese.

Mini Quiches

Hands-On Time: 15 minutes | **Total Time:** 40 minutes plus resting |
Makes: 4 quiches

Quiches are extremely versatile—they work with different vegetables and cheeses, so personalize as you like. Spinach, kale, or Swiss chard can stand in for the arugula; carrots or tomatoes can take the place of the bell pepper. Be sure to cook the vegetables until no liquid remains and then proceed with the recipe. While I love these for breakfast, they would also make a great brown-bag lunch. Wrap each quiche individually in plastic wrap and freeze for up to 3 months. To reheat, wrap in foil and place in the oven at 300°F for about 10 minutes, or thaw overnight in the fridge and serve chilled or at room temperature. This meal is loaded with filling protein (from the eggs and cheese) and soothing omega-3 fats (thanks to the arugula), so you'll never miss the crust!

BELLY BUDDIES:
Olive oil, red bell pepper, arugula, eggs, oat bran

Olive oil spray
- 2 teaspoons extra-virgin olive oil
- 1 small red bell pepper, diced
- 1 bunch arugula (about 4 ounces), coarsely chopped
- 2 large eggs
- 3 large egg whites, or ½ cup liquid egg whites
- 3 tablespoons oat bran
- ½ teaspoon salt
- ¾ cup shredded reduced-fat cheddar cheese (3 ounces)

1. Preheat the oven to 350°F. Coat 4 standard muffin cups with cooking spray.

2. In a medium nonstick skillet, heat the oil over medium heat. Add the bell pepper and cook, stirring occasionally for 7 minutes, or until tender. Add the arugula and cook for 2 minutes, or until wilted.

3. In a large bowl, whisk together the whole eggs, egg whites, oat bran, and salt. Stir in the vegetables and cheese. Spoon the mixture into the muffin cups.

4. Bake for 18 to 20 minutes, or until the eggs are set and the cheese has melted. Let sit for 5 minutes, then run a metal spatula or knife around the edges of the quiches and lift them out of the pan.

5. Serve hot, at room temperature, or chilled.

Per quiche: 187 calories • 13g protein • 10g fat (4.5g saturated) • 2g fiber • 11g carbohydrate • 563mg sodium • 26mg magnesium

If you have gluten issues: Choose a gluten-free brand of oat bran.

Multigrain Hot Cereal with Maple Nuts

Hands-On Time: 20 minutes | **Total Time:** 30 minutes |
Makes: 6 (½-cup) servings

Grain-based hot cereals actually do well if made ahead, refrigerated, and reheated in the microwave. So even if you're cooking for just yourself, make this entire batch and have one portion fresh from the pan. Then refrigerate the rest. Scoop out ½-cup portions as needed, and microwave with a splash of lactose-free milk or coconut milk for 30 to 45 seconds. Soothe your belly with walnuts, which deliver a nice dose of magnesium and omega-3s, two key belly-calming nutrients. Coconut milk is free of lactose so is gentler on your digestive tract. You'll find roasted brown rice couscous in the gluten-free section of most grocery stores.

1 ounce walnuts (generous ¼ cup)

3 tablespoons pure maple syrup

½ cup roasted brown rice couscous

½ cup quinoa, preferably tricolor, rinsed

1 tablespoon chia seeds

½ teaspoon salt

2¼ cups water

1 cup light coconut milk

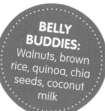
BELLY BUDDIES: Walnuts, brown rice, quinoa, chia seeds, coconut milk

1. In a dry skillet or toaster oven, toast the walnuts for 3 to 5 minutes. While still hot, chop them, place them in a small bowl, and stir in the maple syrup.

2. In a small saucepan, combine the couscous, quinoa, chia seeds, salt, and water. Bring to a boil, then reduce to a simmer, cover, and cook for 8 minutes.

3. Uncover, stir in the coconut milk, and simmer, stirring, for 7 to 9 minutes, or until the grains are tender and the mixture has the consistency of hot cereal.

4. Top each serving of cereal with 2 teaspoons of the maple nuts.

Per serving: 194 calories • 4g protein • 7.5g fat (3g saturated) • 3g fiber • 30g carbohydrate • 203mg sodium • 43mg magnesium

If you have gluten issues: Choose a gluten-free brand of chia seeds.

Toasted Almond Raspberry Muffins

Hands-On Time: 15 minutes | **Total Time:** 40 minutes plus cooling | **Makes:** 12 muffins

These muffins can be made ahead and refrigerated (for up to 7 days) or frozen (for up to 3 months). To freeze, spread the muffins out on a small baking sheet and freeze solid. Then transfer to a resealable plastic freezer bag. Thaw at room temperature. Fiber-rich raspberries keep your intestines moving and your belly flat. Don't use superlarge raspberries for this because they will make the muffins too wet. If you can't find smallish raspberries, then use blueberries instead.

BELLY BUDDIES: Flaxseed, eggs, Greek yogurt, olive oil, raspberries

¾ cup almond flour
1 cup brown rice flour
¼ cup ground flaxseed
2 teaspoons baking powder
1 teaspoon baking soda
½ teaspoon salt
¼ teaspoon ground cardamom

2 large eggs
¾ cup nonfat plain Greek yogurt
½ cup pure maple syrup
3 tablespoons extra-virgin olive oil
6 ounces (about 1½ cups) small raspberries

1. Preheat the oven to 375°F. Line 12 cups of a muffin tin with paper liners.

2. Spread out the almond flour on a baking sheet and bake, stirring once or twice, for 5 to 7 minutes (depending on how thinly you spread the almond flour), or until lightly toasted. Let cool for a minute on the baking sheet, then transfer to a bowl.

3. Add the brown rice flour, flaxseed, baking powder, baking soda, salt, and cardamom to the almond flour and whisk well to combine. With a mixer on low speed, add the eggs, yogurt, maple syrup, and oil and mix until just combined. Fold in the raspberries.

4. Divide the batter among the muffin cups. Bake for 15 to 17 minutes, or until browned on top and a wooden pick inserted in the center of a muffin comes out clean. Cool the muffins on a rack.

Per muffin: 190 calories • 5g protein • 9g fat (1g saturated) • 2.5g fiber • 24g carbohydrate • 317mg sodium • 27mg magnesium

If you have gluten issues: Choose a gluten-free brand of Greek yogurt.

SOUPS

Soothing for your soul and your stomach

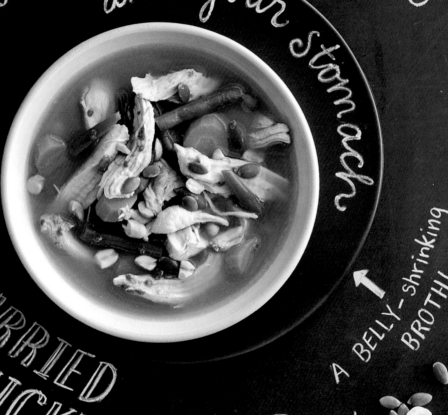

CURRIED CHICKEN SOUP

A BELLY-SHRINKING BROTH!

Curried Chicken Soup

Hands-On Time: 15 minutes | **Total Time:** 35 minutes (plus 30 minutes if making homemade broth) | **Makes:** 4 (1¾-cup) servings

Curry powder, with its key ingredient turmeric, eases inflammation. But check the ingredients: Some curry powders may have onion and/or garlic powder in them. If you plan on using store-bought chicken broth, you could cook the chicken breasts in the simmering broth for 12 minutes, or until cooked through but still a little pink. Let the chicken sit until cool enough to handle, then pull into shreds.

BELLY BUDDIES: Olive oil, chia seeds, carrots, green beans, chicken breast, peanuts, pumpkin seeds

- 1 tablespoon plus 2 teaspoons extra-virgin olive oil
- 2 teaspoons curry powder (onion and garlic free)
- 1 teaspoon chia seeds
- 4 carrots, thinly sliced on an angle
- ½ pound green beans, cut into 1-inch lengths
- ½ teaspoon salt
- 4 cups Homemade Chicken Broth (recipe follows) or store-bought low-sodium chicken broth

- 2 bone-in, skinless chicken breasts (8 ounces each), cooked and shredded (or use the chicken from the Homemade Chicken Broth recipe)
- 2 wedges (¾ ounce each) light spreadable cheese
- 1 tablespoon chopped unsalted peanuts
- 1 tablespoon chopped hulled pumpkin seeds (pepitas)

1. In a large nonstick soup pot or Dutch oven, heat the oil over medium heat. Add the curry powder and chia seeds and cook for 45 seconds, or until fragrant. Add the carrots, green beans, and salt and stir to coat. Add ½ cup of the broth, cover, and simmer for 5 to 7 minutes, or until the carrots are crisp-tender.

2. Add the remaining 3½ cups broth (if you didn't end up with enough broth, just add water) and the chicken and bring back to a simmer. Add the cheese and stir until evenly melted in.

3. Serve in bowls topped with the peanuts and pumpkin seeds.

Per serving: 265 calories • 25g protein • 13g fat (2.5g saturated) • 4g fiber • 13g carbohydrate • 582mg sodium • 60mg magnesium

If you have gluten issues: Choose gluten-free brands of curry powder, chia seeds, chicken broth, and light spreadable cheese.

Homemade Chicken Broth

To make a double batch of this broth, add 1 more chicken breast (save it for a lunch salad), double the water you use, add at least 1 more carrot and 1 more celery rib, and double the herbs. Free of onion and garlic, your belly will thank you for the extra effort of making this soothing, belly-shrinking broth.

2 bone-in, skinless chicken breasts (8 ounces each)

2 carrots, cut into 1-inch chunks

2 small ribs celery, cut into 1-inch chunks

½ small lemon, sliced

½ teaspoon black peppercorns

4 scallion greens

2 or 3 large sprigs parsley

2 small sprigs thyme

1 bay leaf

8 cups water

¼ teaspoon salt

1. In a large saucepan, combine the chicken, carrots, celery, lemon, peppercorns, scallion greens, parsley, thyme, and bay leaf. Add the water and bring to a boil over high heat. Add the salt, reduce to a simmer, and cook for 12 minutes, or until the chicken is cooked through but still a little pink.

2. Remove the chicken, but keep the broth at a low simmer. When the chicken is cool enough to handle, pull the meat off the bones and return the bones to the simmering broth. Let the broth simmer for 30 minutes longer to develop flavor (this step is optional, but will make a much more flavorful broth). Strain the broth and discard the solids.

Caldo Verde

Hands-On Time: 15 minutes | **Total Time:** 30 minutes | **Makes:** 4 (2-cup) servings

Caldo Verde is a traditional Portuguese greens soup that is made with a garlicky sausage seasoned with paprika and wine. Here we've replicated some of those flavors but without all the fat and garlic. You can make the soup ahead and refrigerate for up to 4 days, but don't freeze it because the potatoes will get spongy. This kale-rich soup provides a nice dose of the anti-inflammation powerhouse magnesium!

BELLY BUDDIES: Olive oil, turnips, potatoes, kale, lemon

- 1 tablespoon plus 1 teaspoon Roasted Garlic Oil (page 211) or extra-virgin olive oil
- 4 ounces all-natural uncured smoked ham, cut into slivers
- 2 teaspoons hot paprika
- ¾ cup dry white wine
- 5 cups low-sodium chicken broth
- ¾ pound white turnips (2 medium), cut into ½-inch cubes
- ¾ pound red potatoes (2 medium), cut into ½-inch cubes
- ¼ teaspoon salt
- 6 cups packed shredded kale leaves (from an 8-ounce bunch)

Lemon wedges

1. In a large nonstick Dutch oven, heat the oil over medium-high heat. Add the ham, sprinkle with paprika, and cook for 2 to 3 minutes, or until starting to crisp. Stir in the wine and simmer for 1 minute to cook off some of the alcohol.

2. Add the broth, turnips, potatoes, and salt and bring to a boil. Add the kale a handful at a time, stirring and adding more as it wilts into the soup. Partially cover the pot and simmer for 10 to 15 minutes, or until the kale, potatoes, and turnips are all tender. Ladle into a bowl and squeeze a lemon wedge over top.

Per serving: 262 calories • 15g protein • 6.5g fat (1g saturated) • 5.5g fiber • 32g carbohydrate • 511mg sodium • 64mg magnesium

If you have gluten issues: Choose gluten-free brands of hot paprika and chicken broth.

Creamy Chard and Spinach Soup

Hands-On Time: 25 minutes | **Total Time:** 35 minutes | **Makes:** 4 (2-cup) servings

Both almond butter and ⅓-less-fat cream cheese give a rich finish to the soup, as does pureeing some of the greens. This is the perfect place to use an immersion blender if you have one. Swiss chard is rich in anti-inflammatory antioxidants, which soothe your digestive tract.

- 1 tablespoon extra-virgin olive oil
- 1 red bell pepper, diced
- ½ cup sliced scallion greens or chives
- ¾ pound Swiss chard, leaves and stems thinly sliced (6 cups)
- 2 packages (10 ounces each) frozen chopped spinach, thawed
- 3 cups low-sodium chicken broth
- 2½ cups water
- ½ teaspoon salt
- 3 tablespoons natural almond butter
- 2 tablespoons (1 ounce) ⅓-less-fat cream cheese

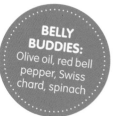

BELLY BUDDIES: Olive oil, red bell pepper, Swiss chard, spinach

1. In a large saucepan, heat the oil over medium-low heat. Add the bell pepper and scallion greens and cook, stirring occasionally, for 7 minutes, or until the pepper is crisp-tender.

2. Add the chard and cook for 1 minute, or until wilted. Add the spinach, broth, water, and salt and bring to a boil over medium heat. Reduce to a simmer and cook, uncovered, for 5 minutes, or until the chard and spinach are very tender.

3. Add the almond butter and cream cheese and cook for 1 minute, or until they've melted and the soup is lightly thickened. Transfer 2 cups of the soup to a blender or food processor and puree. Stir it back into the soup, gently reheating if necessary. Serve hot.

Per serving: 195 calories • 11g protein • 13g fat (2g saturated) • 7g fiber • 13g carbohydrate • 589mg sodium • 190mg magnesium

If you have gluten issues: Choose a gluten-free brand of chicken broth.

Hearty Roasted Vegetable Soup

Hands-On Time: 20 minutes | **Total Time:** 1 hour | **Makes:** 4 (2-cup) servings

Roasting the vegetables brings out their natural sugars and makes for a richer, more deeply flavored soup. The vegetables are roasted on a rimmed baking sheet (like a jelly-roll pan) rather than a roasting pan, as the low walls allow better air circulation and the vegetables will roast and brown instead of steam. If you don't have one, use a large baking sheet, but just be careful when you're tossing the vegetables. This fiber-rich soup will soothe and trim your belly fat by cooling inflammation.

BELLY BUDDIES: Tomatoes, potatoes, green beans, carrot, parsnips, olive oil, almonds

1½ pounds plum tomatoes, cut into 1-inch chunks

1 pound russet (baking) potatoes, peeled, quartered, and thinly sliced

¾ pound green beans, cut into 1-inch lengths

1 large carrot (8 ounces), thinly sliced

2 small parsnips (6 ounces total), thinly sliced

4 scallion greens, thinly sliced (½ cup)

1 tablespoon plus 1 teaspoon extra-virgin olive oil

4 cups water

1 teaspoon dried basil

½ teaspoon salt

¼ teaspoon black pepper

⅔ cup grated Parmesan cheese

½ cup sliced almonds

1. Preheat the oven to 425°F. On a large rimmed baking sheet, toss together the tomatoes, potatoes, green beans, carrot, parsnips, scallion greens, and oil. Roast, turning the vegetables occasionally, for 30 minutes, or until lightly browned and crisp-tender.

2. Transfer the vegetables and any juices on the baking sheet to a large saucepan. Add the water, basil, salt, and pepper and bring to a boil over high heat. Reduce to a simmer and cook, uncovered, for 10 minutes, or until the vegetables are tender.

3. Ladle the soup into bowls and top with the cheese and nuts.

Per serving: 368 calories • 14g protein • 15g fat (3.5g saturated) • 11g fiber • 50g carbohydrate • 559mg sodium • 125mg magnesium

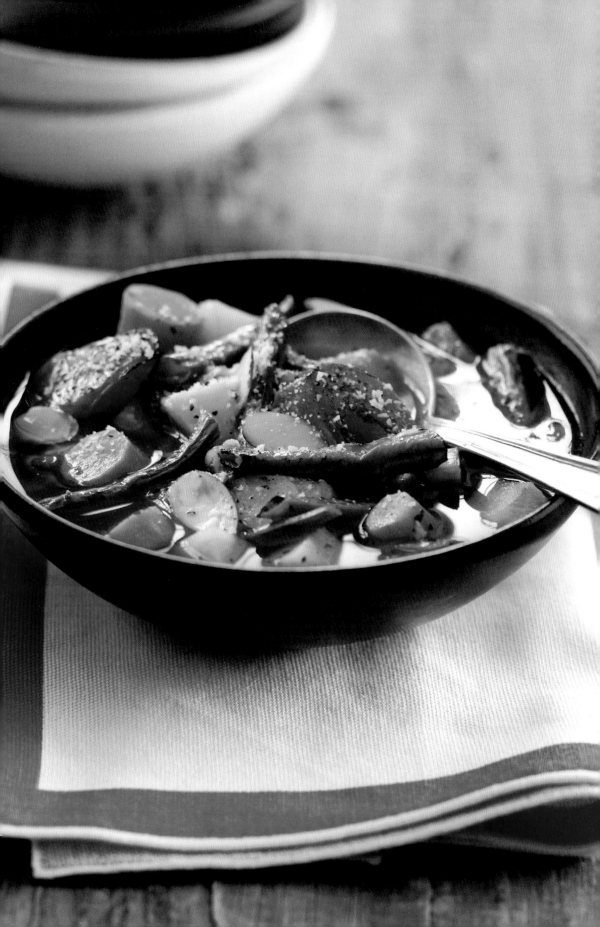

MAIN COURSES

CROWD-PLEASING ENTRÉES
TO TRIM AND TAME YOUR TUMMY

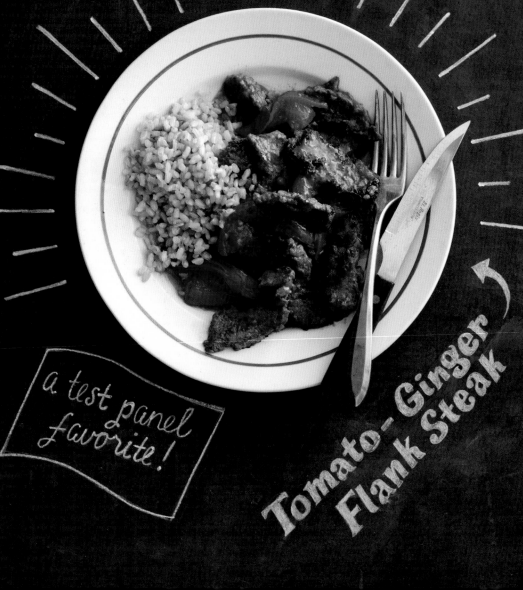

a test panel
favorite!

Tomato-Ginger
Flank Steak

Tomato-Ginger Flank Steak

Hands-On Time: 15 minutes | **Total Time:** 45 minutes | **Makes:** 4 (1-cup) servings

The steak and tomatoes produce a fair amount of "sauce," so if you're having this on Phase 2, serve with ½ cup cooked quinoa, and on Phase 3, serve with ½ cup cooked brown rice. Start the meal with a simple tossed salad (at least 2 cups of greens per person, tossed with a light vinaigrette: 1 part vinegar to 1 part extra-virgin olive oil). Ginger infuses wonderful flavor while easing inflammation and aiding digestion.

1¼ pounds flank steak

2 tablespoons grated fresh ginger

1 teaspoon ground ginger

½ teaspoon salt

4 teaspoons extra-virgin olive oil

4 plum tomatoes (about 1 pound), cut into thin wedges

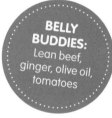

BELLY BUDDIES: Lean beef, ginger, olive oil, tomatoes

1. Cut the steak with the grain (lengthwise) into thirds, then cut each piece crosswise (across the grain) into very thin slices. Place in a bowl. Add the fresh ginger, ground ginger, salt, and 2 teaspoons of the oil. Toss the steak well to coat and let sit at room temperature for 30 minutes.

2. In a large nonstick skillet, heat the remaining 2 teaspoons oil over medium-high heat. Add the steak and cook, tossing to get all sides of the slices, for 1 to 2 minutes, or until a little browned but still quite pink. Transfer the steak to a plate.

3. Add the tomatoes to the skillet and cook for 1 minute to heat through. Return the steak (and any juices from the plate) to the skillet and toss well to combine. Cook for 1 to 2 minutes, or until the tomatoes have collapsed a bit and the steak is hot.

Per serving: 264 calories • 32g protein • 13g fat (3.5g saturated) • 1.5g fiber • 5g carbohydrate • 375mg sodium • 47mg magnesium

Test Team Fave!

"My son's scout troop made tomato ginger flank steak for dinner. We grilled outside in the snow and had a blast. There was no steak left over! On another night I fed my whole family ginger flank steak and it was a huge hit. My wife even commented that it was delicious cold over salad. For me it was a great meal: not a lot of ingredients, simple steps, and easy clean up." —JONATHAN BIGHAM

Grilled Turkey Cutlets with Grape Salsa

Hands-On Time: 15 minutes | **Total Time:** 15 minutes | **Makes:** 4 servings

Take this supersimple salsa and swap in different fruits. You need to stay with something of similar texture and sweet-tart balance. Try pineapple, kiwi, blueberries, or grape tomatoes (remember, a tomato is a fruit, too!). Serve the turkey and salsa with boiled red potatoes (1 medium or 3 small per person) and steamed green beans or wilted kale.

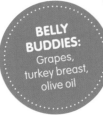

BELLY BUDDIES: Grapes, turkey breast, olive oil

6 ounces red grapes (about 12 large), coarsely chopped

1 teaspoon fresh lime juice

Large pinch of cayenne pepper

Coarse (kosher) salt

2 tablespoons chopped fresh cilantro

4 turkey breast cutlets or steaks (4 ounces each, about ½ inch thick)

1 tablespoon plus 1 teaspoon extra-virgin olive oil

Black pepper

1. In a bowl, combine the grapes, lime juice, cayenne, and a pinch of salt. Let sit for at least 15 minutes. Just before serving, stir in the cilantro.

2. Preheat a grill pan or grill to medium-high. Coat both sides of the turkey with the oil. Sprinkle both sides with a pinch of salt and pepper.

3. Grill the turkey for 3 minutes on one side, then flip and cook for 2 minutes, or until cooked through but still juicy.

4. Serve topped with the grape salsa.

Per serving: 190 calories • 28g protein • 6g fat (0.5g saturated) • 0.5g fiber • 8g carbohydrate • 126mg sodium • 3mg magnesium

Kiwi-Glazed Turkey Meat Loaf

Hands-On Time: 15 minutes | **Total Time:** 1 hour plus cooling | **Makes:** 6 servings

When you make meat loaves with very lean cuts of meat or poultry, it helps to line the loaf pan with parchment paper to prevent sticking. As a bonus, with the overhang, you can lift the meat loaf out and not have to struggle to get out that first slice. Peanut butter is rich in protein and the anti-inflammation belly soothers monounsaturated fats and magnesium. Serve the meat loaf with Crunchy Chopped Salad (page 202).

⅓ cup brown rice couscous
¼ teaspoon ground coriander
¾ teaspoon salt
2 kiwis
¼ cup natural peanut butter
2 large eggs

1¼ pounds ground turkey breast
1 red bell pepper, diced
½ cup chopped fresh cilantro
¼ cup ground flaxseed
¼ teaspoon black pepper

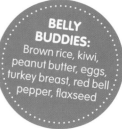

BELLY BUDDIES: Brown rice, kiwi, peanut butter, eggs, turkey breast, red bell pepper, flaxseed

1. Preheat the oven to 350°F. Line the bottom and long sides of a 9 x 5-inch loaf pan with parchment paper (leave some overhang at the top so you can lift the meat loaf out).

2. In a small saucepan, cook the couscous according to package directions using the coriander and ¼ teaspoon of the salt. Transfer the couscous to a plate, fluffing it with a fork.

3. Meanwhile, halve the kiwis and use a spoon to scoop out and discard the center core and the seeds (don't try to get all the seeds, just most of them). Scoop the kiwi flesh out of the skins into a mini food processor and puree until smooth.

4. In a small glass bowl, heat the peanut butter in the microwave to make it liquidy, cooking it in 10-second increments and stirring after each. Let cool slightly, then beat in the eggs.

5. In a large bowl, combine the turkey, peanut butter mixture, couscous, bell pepper, cilantro, flaxseed, black pepper, and the remaining ½ teaspoon salt and mix well. Mound into the loaf pan and spread the kiwi puree over the top.

6. Bake for 45 minutes, or until firm and cooked through. Let rest 15 minutes before lifting out and slicing.

Per serving: 266 calories • 30g protein • 10g fat (1g saturated) • 4g fiber • 16g carbohydrate • 362mg sodium • 8mg magnesium

Curry-Rubbed Chicken with Fresh Pineapple Chutney

Hands-On Time: 10 minutes | **Total Time:** 40 minutes | **Makes:** 4 servings

Cooking chicken breast on the bone and with its skin helps it stay juicy, but because the skin doesn't get eaten, the flavorings here are rubbed under the skin right onto the chicken flesh. Instead of taking the chicken off the bone as directed, you could serve it bone-in. Enjoy the chicken with a side of Creamed Spinach (page 212) or steamed greens.

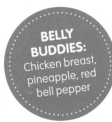

BELLY BUDDIES: Chicken breast, pineapple, red bell pepper

1½ teaspoons curry powder (onion and garlic free)

½ teaspoon coarse (kosher) salt

½ teaspoon ground cinnamon

4 bone-in, skin-on chicken breast halves (10 ounces each)

1 cup diced fresh pineapple

1 small red bell pepper, diced

1 tablespoon pure maple syrup

1 tablespoon coconut oil, melted

2 teaspoons red wine vinegar

1. Preheat the oven to 375°F.

2. In a small bowl, combine the curry powder, salt, and cinnamon. With your fingers, carefully lift the skin of the chicken and rub the curry mixture on the meat. Pull the skin back over the chicken.

3. Place the chicken on a rimmed baking sheet or on a small roasting pan and roast for 30 minutes, or until just cooked through. When cool enough to handle, remove the skin.

4. Meanwhile, in a small bowl, combine the pineapple, bell pepper, maple syrup, oil, and vinegar.

5. Cut the chicken off the bone, slice, and serve with the pineapple chutney.

Per serving: 291 calories • 42g protein • 8.5g fat (4.5g saturated) • 1.5g fiber • 11g carbohydrate • 341mg sodium • 49mg magnesium

If you have gluten issues: Choose a gluten-free brand of curry powder.

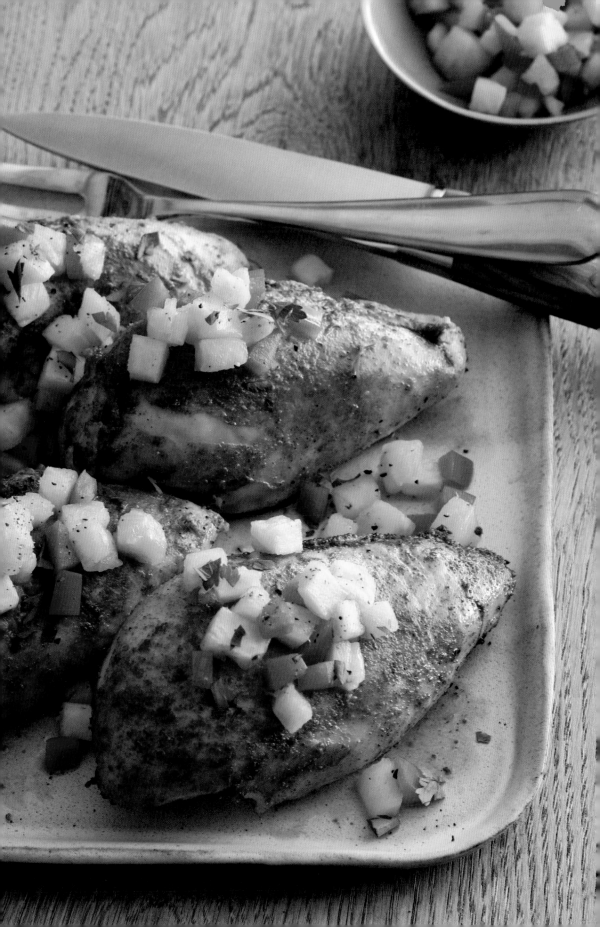

Arugula Pesto Chicken

Hands-On Time: 15 minutes | **Total Time:** 40 minutes | Makes: 4 servings

For a "fancy" presentation, you could slice the chicken so that the pesto shows. If you plan on doing that, let the chicken rest for at least 5 minutes before you slice it. If you're on Phase 3, serve this with Toasted Brown Rice and Pepper Pilaf (page 222). If you're on Phases 1 or 2, serve with Twice-Baked Potato with Pepper Hash (page 219). This recipe provides key inflammation-fighting fats (monounsaturated fats and omega-3s) to calm and ease your digestive system.

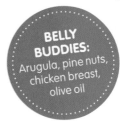

BELLY BUDDIES:
Arugula, pine nuts, chicken breast, olive oil

- 1 cup packed baby arugula (1 ounce)
- 3 tablespoons pine nuts or slivered almonds, toasted
- ¼ cup grated Parmesan cheese
- 2 tablespoons water

- 4 boneless, skinless chicken breast halves (6 ounces each)
- 1 tablespoon extra-virgin olive oil
- ½ teaspoon ground cumin
- 4 pinches of coarse (kosher) salt

1. Preheat the oven to 400°F

2. In a mini food processor, combine the arugula, pine nuts, Parmesan, and water. Grind to a coarse paste.

3. With a sharp knife, make a horizontal cut into the flesh on the flat, smooth side of a chicken breast. Wiggle the knife around to make a pocket in the chicken (taking care not to cut through to the other side). Stuff each chicken breast with 2 tablespoons of the pesto. Press the chicken closed.

4. Pour the oil into a 7 x 11-inch baking dish. One by one, put the chicken in, smooth side down, to coat with a little oil. Then flip and place in the oil, smooth side up. Sprinkle the tops of the chicken with the cumin and salt.

5. Bake for 25 minutes, or until the chicken is cooked through but still juicy. Serve the chicken with some of the pan juices drizzled on top.

Per serving: 290 calories • 39g protein • 14g fat (2.5g saturated) • 0.5g fiber • 1g carbohydrate • 396mg sodium • 64mg magnesium

Tuna Romesco

Hands-On Time: 10 minutes │ **Total Time:** 15 minutes │ **Makes:** 4 servings

Tuna is rich in belly-soothing omega-3 fats. Like steak, it can be cooked to any degree of doneness. The timing given here will result in medium to medium-rare doneness. The sauce (based on a Spanish sauce typically used for grilled vegetables) can be made several days ahead and stored in the refrigerator. You can make this into a great salad: Thinly slice the cooked tuna and toss it with the romesco sauce and 1½ cups cooked green beans. Or serve the tuna with steamed green beans or Green Beans Amandine (page 214).

1 large roasted red bell pepper (from a jar or a salad bar)

½ cup canned no-salt-added crushed tomatoes (look for brands with no onions or garlic)

¼ cup water

2 tablespoons raw (skin-on) almonds

¾ teaspoon paprika

½ teaspoon salt

4 teaspoons extra-virgin olive oil

4 tuna steaks (5 ounces each)

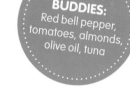

BELLY BUDDIES: Red bell pepper, tomatoes, almonds, olive oil, tuna

1. In a food processor, combine the bell pepper, tomatoes, water, almonds, paprika, salt, and 2 teaspoons of the oil and puree until smooth.

2. In a large nonstick skillet, heat the remaining 2 teaspoons oil over medium heat. Add the tuna and cook for 2 minutes per side, or until lightly crisped on the outside and still pink inside.

3. Serve the tuna with the sauce spooned over the top.

Per serving: 288 calories • 35g protein • 14g fat (2.5g saturated) • 2g fiber • 4g carbohydrate • 392mg sodium • 92mg magnesium

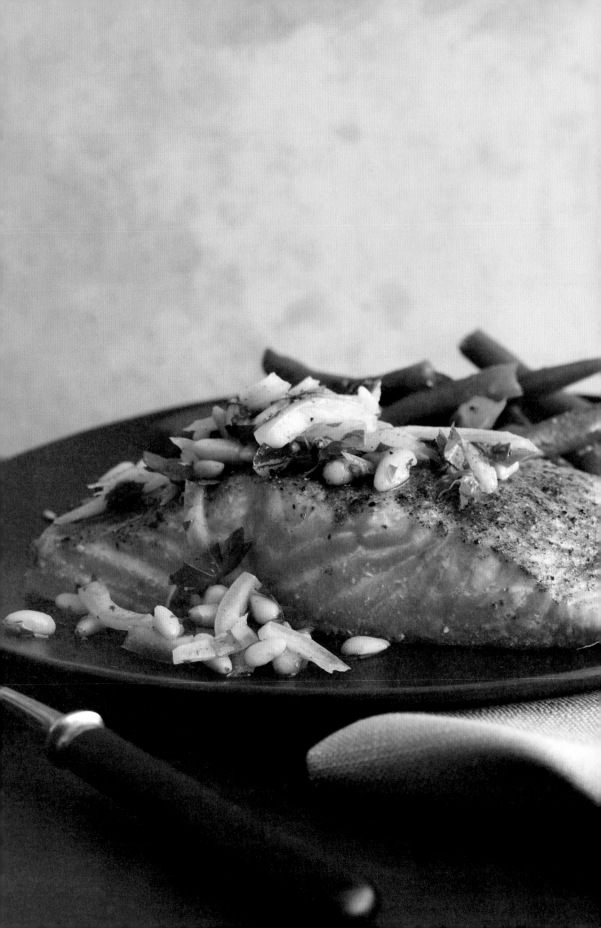

Salmon with Preserved Lemon Topping

Hands-On Time: 20 minutes | **Total Time:** 20 minutes | **Makes:** 4 servings

Preserved lemons, a staple in North African cooking, take several weeks to make, but here is a super-quick method for getting the same flavors in under 30 minutes. The lemon relish, which is spiced with a little garam masala (an Indian spice blend), makes a pleasantly astringent topping for the rich salmon. Serve with Green Beans Amandine (page 214) or, in Phase 2, Summer Squash Gratin (page 215) or Nutty Red Quinoa (page 220).

- 1 lemon
- ½ teaspoon coarse (kosher) salt
- 4 skin-on salmon fillets (5 ounces each)
- 1¼ teaspoons garam masala
- 1 tablespoon fresh lemon juice
- 1 teaspoon slivered almonds or pine nuts
- 1 teaspoon extra-virgin olive oil
- 1 tablespoon water
- 1 tablespoon chopped fresh parsley

BELLY BUDDIES: Lemon, salmon, almonds, olive oil

1. Preheat the oven to 450°F.

2. With a vegetable peeler, pull off all the lemon zest in strips. In a small saucepan of boiling water, cook the zest for 2 minutes to blanch. Drain and repeat the blanching in new water. Drain again. Rinse under cold water and drain well. Coarsely chop and transfer to a small bowl. Sprinkle with ¼ teaspoon of the salt and let stand while the salmon roasts.

3. Place the salmon, skin side down, on a rimmed baking sheet and rub with 1 teaspoon of the garam masala and the remaining ¼ teaspoon salt. Roast for 10 minutes, or until the salmon is just cooked through. Using a thin-bladed metal spatula, lift the salmon off the baking sheet, leaving the skin behind.

4. Drain any liquid from the bowl with the lemon zest. Add the lemon juice, almonds, oil, water, parsley, and the remaining ¼ teaspoon garam masala to the bowl and toss to combine.

5. Serve the salmon with the lemon mixture on top.

Per serving: 268 calories • 27g protein • 16g fat (3g saturated) • 1.5g fiber • 3g carbohydrate • 315mg sodium • 42mg magnesium

If you have gluten issues: Choose a gluten-free brand of garam masala.

Paprika-Spiced Fish Cakes

Hands-On Time: 25 minutes | **Total Time:** 1 hour 10 minutes | **Makes:** 4 servings

To make ahead, you can form the fish cakes and freeze: Place the cakes on a baking sheet or platter and freeze solid. Once frozen, wrap each individually, transfer to a resealable plastic bag, and keep in the freezer for up to 3 months. You can serve these at a moment's notice, because you can actually cook them straight from frozen. To do that, brown the cakes as directed in the recipe, but then transfer them to a 350°F oven and bake for 5 minutes, or until piping hot. Serve with Creamed Spinach (page 212).

BELLY BUDDIES: Potatoes, fish, oat bran, egg, lemon, olive oil

- 10 ounces russet (baking) potatoes, peeled and thinly sliced
- 1 pound skinless grouper or cod fillets, cut into large chunks
- 3 tablespoons oat bran
- 1 large egg
- 2 tablespoons fresh lemon juice
- 1½ teaspoons smoked paprika
- ½ teaspoon salt
- ¼ teaspoon black pepper
- ½ cup thinly sliced scallion greens
- 4 teaspoons Roasted Garlic Oil (page 211) or extra-virgin olive oil

Lemon wedges (optional)

1. Place the potatoes in a medium saucepan and cover with cold water. Bring to a boil and cook for 12 minutes, or until the potatoes are tender. Drain well. Transfer to a large bowl and mash with a potato masher or handheld mixer. Cool to room temperature.

2. In a food processor, combine the fish, oat bran, egg, lemon juice, paprika, salt, and pepper. Pulse until the fish is finely ground.

3. Transfer the mixture to the bowl with the potatoes. Add the scallion greens and mix well to combine. Using a ½-cup measuring cup, scoop the mixture and shape into 8 fish cakes. Transfer to a platter and refrigerate for 30 minutes.

4. In a large nonstick or cast-iron skillet, heat 2 teaspoons of the oil over medium heat. Add half the fish cakes and cook for 3 minutes, or until browned. Flip the fish cakes over and cook for 3 minutes, or until browned. Repeat with the remaining 2 teaspoons oil and the 4 remaining fish cakes.

5. Serve 2 fish cakes per person, with lemon wedges, if desired.

Per serving: 235 calories • 26g protein • 7.5g fat (1.5g saturated) • 2g fiber • 17g carbohydrate • 373mg sodium • 68mg magnesium

If you have gluten issues: Choose gluten-free brands of oat bran and paprika.

Chipotle Veggie Burgers

Hands-On Time: 15 minutes | **Total Time:** 30 minutes | **Makes:** 4 burgers

Vinegar, chipotle chile powder, and oregano combine with a little tomato paste to replicate the flavors of chiles in adobo sauce, but without all the garlic and onion. (While tomato paste contains some FODMAPs, the amount here is small enough that it won't bother your tummy.) Serve the burgers on a bed of lettuce with Summer Squash Gratin (page 215) and sliced tomatoes.

- 2 tablespoons no-salt-added tomato paste
- 1 tablespoon red wine vinegar
- ¼ to ½ teaspoon chipotle chile powder
- ¼ teaspoon dried oregano
- ⅓ cup dry kasha (roasted buckwheat groats)
- ½ teaspoon salt
- 1 medium zucchini (8 ounces)
- ⅓ cup finely chopped pecans
- 1 large egg
- 1 large egg white
- 1 tablespoon plus 1 teaspoon extra-virgin olive oil
- 2 ounces sliced reduced-fat smoked provolone (or other reduced-fat cheese), cut to fit the tops of the burgers

BELLY BUDDIES: Tomatoes, zucchini, pecans, egg, olive oil

1. In a small bowl, combine the tomato paste, vinegar, chipotle powder (to taste), and oregano. Measure out 1 tablespoon and mix with 2 teaspoons water in a cup.

2. In a small saucepan, cook the kasha according to package directions with ½ teaspoon salt. Drain very well and spread out on a plate lined with paper towel to cool.

3. Shred the zucchini on the medium holes of a box grater over a kitchen towel. Twist the zucchini up in the towel and wring out as much moisture as you can. Transfer the zucchini to a large bowl.

4. Add the cooled kasha, pecans, whole egg, egg white, and the remaining tomato paste mixture to the zucchini and stir well to blend. Pack the mixture into a ½-cup measure to make 4 cakes, inverting them onto a plate. Refrigerate for 30 minutes to firm up a little.

5. In a large nonstick skillet, heat the oil over medium-high heat. Add the burgers and cook for 3 minutes without turning. Carefully turn, reduce the heat to medium, top with the reserved tomato paste mixture, and cook for 5 to 7 minutes, or until the second side is browned and the burgers are heated through.

6. Turn off the heat, top the burgers with the cheese, cover the pan, and let sit for 3 minutes to melt the cheese.

Per burger: 235 calories • 10g protein • 16g fat (3.5g saturated) • 3g fiber • 16g carbohydrate • 135mg sodium • 58mg magnesium

Ratatouille Frittata

Hands-On Time: 15 minutes | **Total Time:** 55 minutes plus cooling | **Makes:** 4 servings

If you have a medium nonstick skillet (10 inches) that can go in the oven, use it here to get thicker frittata wedges. The stove-top time for setting the eggs will be the same, but the time in the oven will be a bit longer. Check the frittata at the 25- or 30-minute mark, and then set your timer to check several times over the next 5 to 10 minutes. Serve the frittata with baby spinach tossed with a garlic-lemon vinaigrette (1 part Roasted Garlic Oil, page 211, to 1 part lemon juice).

BELLY BUDDIES:
Potato, eggs, olive oil, zucchini, eggplants, tomatoes

- 1 medium Yukon Gold potato (6 ounces), cut into ½-inch cubes
- 6 large eggs
- 5 large egg whites (or ¾ cup liquid egg whites)
- 1 teaspoon dried tarragon
- ¼ teaspoon black pepper
- ½ teaspoon salt
- 1 tablespoon plus 1 teaspoon extra-virgin olive oil

- 1 medium zucchini (8 ounces), cut into ½-inch cubes
- 2 baby Italian eggplants (5 ounces each), cut into ½-inch cubes
- 2 plum tomatoes, cut into ½-inch cubes
- 6 tablespoons grated Parmesan cheese

1. Preheat the oven to 350°F.

2. In a steamer, cook the potato for 5 to 7 minutes, or until tender.

3. In a large bowl, beat together the whole eggs, egg whites, tarragon, pepper, and ¼ teaspoon of the salt.

4. In a large nonstick ovenproof skillet, heat the oil over medium-high heat. Add the zucchini and cook for 2 minutes, or until beginning to soften. Add the eggplant, sprinkle with the remaining ¼ teaspoon salt, and cook without stirring for 3 minutes. Add the tomatoes and stir to combine. Cover and cook for 3 minutes, or until the eggplant is mostly tender and the tomatoes have given up some liquid.

5. Add the potatoes and toss to coat. Pour the eggs over the pan and cook for 2 minutes, or until the edges are just starting to set. Sprinkle with the Parmesan and transfer to the oven. Bake for 25 to 30 minutes, or until the frittata is set, puffed, and browned. Let stand for 5 minutes before cutting.

Per serving: 264 calories • 19g protein • 14g fat (4.5g saturated) • 4g fiber • 15g carbohydrate • 596mg sodium • 50mg magnesium

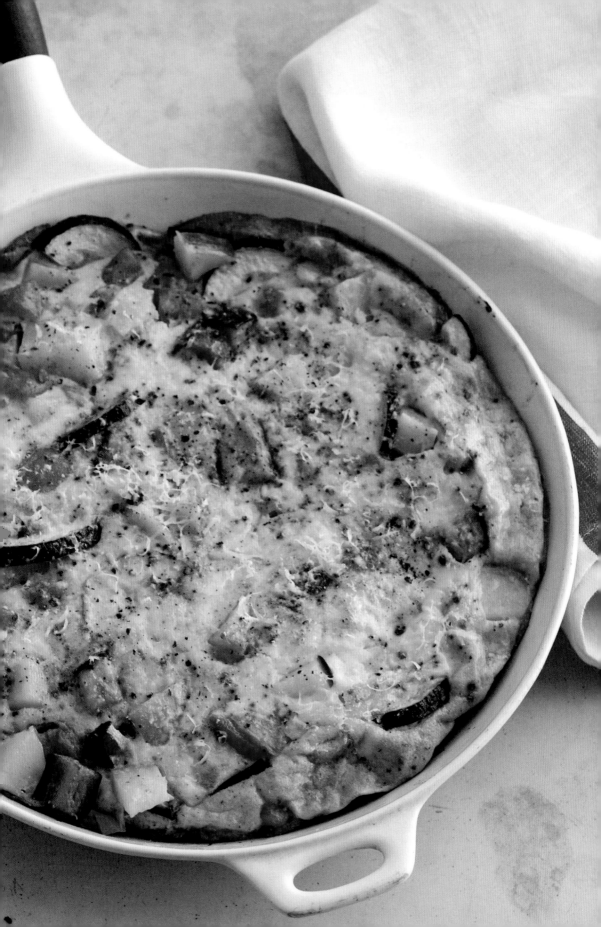

ONE-DISH MAINS

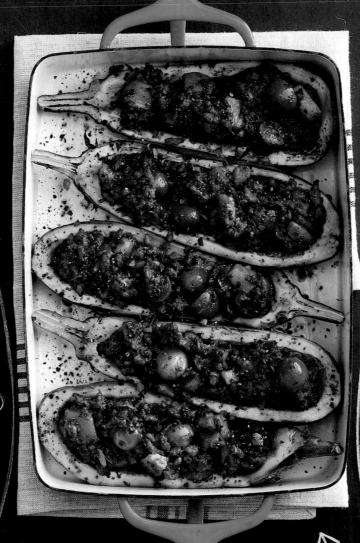

Hearty all-in-one meals

to slim and calm your belly

BEEF & QUINOA
STUFFED EGGPLANT

Beef and Red Quinoa–Stuffed Eggplant

Hands-On Time: 25 minutes | **Total Time:** 55 minutes | **Makes:** 4 servings

If you can't find small eggplants, swap in 2 larger ones, about 1 pound each. The cooking times should be about the same. When shopping for eggplants, look for those that are firm and shiny, without any soft spots. Both the filling and the eggplants can be made ahead and refrigerated separately. Or the eggplants can be filled a day ahead, refrigerated, and baked when ready to serve. This satisfying recipe includes lots of belly-friendly fiber to keep you full, while chia seeds provide an extra kick of omega-3 fats for a soothing boost.

- 4 small eggplants (8 ounces each)
- 1¾ cups water
- 2 teaspoons extra-virgin olive oil
- ½ cup red quinoa
- ¾ pound 93% lean ground beef
- ½ teaspoon ground cinnamon
- ¾ teaspoon salt
- 1 cup canned no-salt-added crushed tomatoes (look for brands with no onions or garlic)
- 20 red seedless grapes, halved
- 1 tablespoon chia seeds

BELLY BUDDIES: Eggplant, olive oil, quinoa, lean beef, tomatoes, grapes, chia seeds

1. Preheat the oven to 400°F. Halve each eggplant lengthwise. With a paring knife, cut around the edge of the eggplants, leaving a ½-inch border, and cut out the flesh of the eggplants. Dice the eggplant flesh.

2. Place the eggplant shells, cut side down, on a rimmed baking sheet. Pour ½ cup of the water onto the baking sheet and bake for 15 minutes, or until the shells are tender.

3. Meanwhile, in a large nonstick skillet, heat the oil over medium-low heat. Add the eggplant flesh and ¼ cup of the water and cook for 2 minutes. Add the quinoa, beef, cinnamon, and salt and cook, stirring, for 3 minutes, or until the beef is no longer pink. Add the tomatoes and the remaining 1 cup water and bring to a boil.

4. Reduce to a simmer, cover, and cook for 15 minutes, or until the quinoa is tender. Stir in the grapes.

5. Turn the eggplant shells cut side up and divide the quinoa mixture among them. Bake for 10 minutes, or until piping hot. Sprinkle with the chia seeds and serve hot or at room temperature.

Per serving: 342 calories • 24g protein • 12g fat (3g saturated) • 11g fiber • 37g carbohydrate • 447mg sodium • 59mg magnesium

If you have gluten issues: Choose a gluten-free brand of chia seeds.

Pork Satay Salad

Hands-On Time: 20 minutes | **Total Time:** 55 minutes | **Makes:** 4 (3-cup) servings

A satay is a Southeast Asian dish that typically involves grilled meat kebabs served with a peanut sauce. Here the pork is roasted whole before slicing, and the peanut sauce becomes a salad dressing. The pork can be made up to 2 days ahead, the dressing up to a week ahead, and the fruit cut up, but don't combine all the ingredients until ready to serve. The papaya contains an enzyme (called papain) that causes protein to break down—in fact, it's the main ingredient in some meat tenderizers.

BELLY BUDDIES:
Lean pork, olive oil, peanut butter, papaya, oranges, lettuce, endive

- 1 pound pork tenderloin
- ½ teaspoon mild to medium chili powder (onion and garlic free)
- ¾ teaspoon coarse (kosher) salt
- 3 teaspoons extra-virgin olive oil
- 2 tablespoons natural peanut butter, at room temperature
- 2 tablespoons fresh lime juice
- 4 cups 2-inch-wide romaine lettuce strips
- 1 Belgian endive, halved lengthwise and thinly sliced crosswise
- 2 cups 1-inch papaya chunks
- 2 navel oranges, peeled and cut into segments

1. Preheat the oven to 400°F. Place the pork on a rimmed baking sheet and rub with the chili powder, ½ teaspoon of the salt, and 1 teaspoon of the oil. Roast the pork for 25 to 30 minutes, or until an instant-read thermometer inserted in the thickest part of the pork registers 145°F. Let the pork rest for 10 minutes before thinly slicing.

2. Meanwhile, in a small bowl, whisk together the peanut butter, lime juice, the remaining 2 teaspoons oil, and the remaining ¼ teaspoon salt.

3. On a large plate, layer the romaine, endive, papaya, orange segments, and pork. Drizzle with the dressing and serve immediately.

Per serving: 279 calories • 25g protein • 11g fat (2g saturated) • 5g fiber • 21g carbohydrate • 423mg sodium • 56mg magnesium

If you have gluten issues: Choose a gluten-free brand of chili powder.

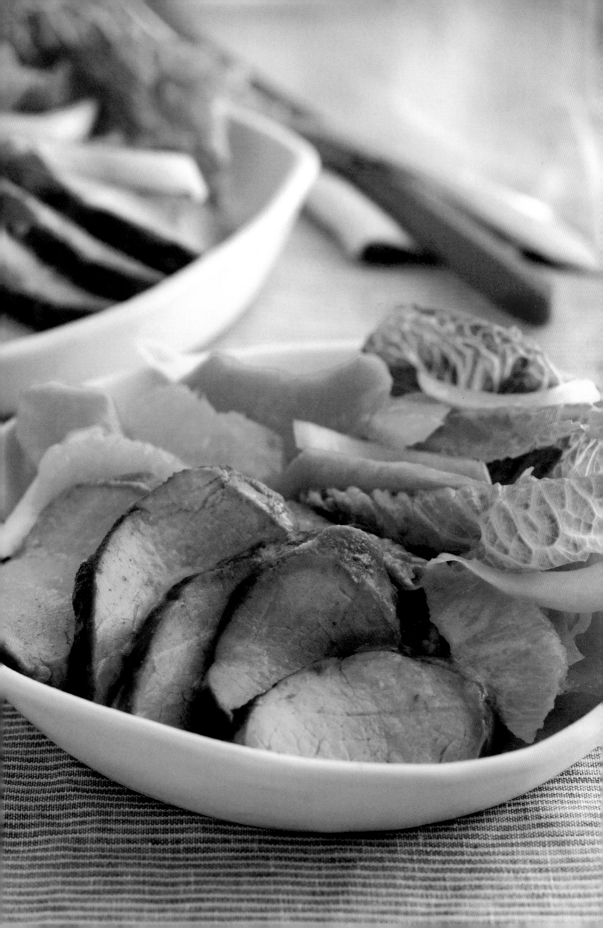

Baked Pork Tetrazzini

Hands-On Time: 20 minutes | **Total Time:** 55 minutes | **Makes:** 6 servings

Rutabaga, a yellow turnip, is a nutrient-rich root loaded with potassium, vitamin C, and fiber. Serve this with a simple tossed salad, such as Butter Lettuce with Scallion-Ginger Vinaigrette (page 203).

BELLY BUDDIES: Olive oil, rutabaga, pork loin, brown rice pasta, red bell pepper

Olive oil spray

Salt

8 ounces brown rice spaghetti or linguine, broken into 2-inch pieces

½ teaspoon ground cumin

½ teaspoon smoked paprika

1 medium-large rutabaga (12 ounces), peeled and cut into ½-inch cubes

1 pound boneless pork loin chops, cut into ½-inch cubes

4 teaspoons olive oil

1 red bell pepper, diced

¼ cup brown rice flour

1½ cups lactose-free 1% milk

8 tablespoons grated Parmesan cheese

Black pepper

1. Preheat the oven to 375°F. Lightly coat the bottom and sides of a 9 x 13-inch baking dish with olive oil spray.

2. Bring a large pot of water to a boil. Add 1 teaspoon salt to the water, then add the pasta and cook for two-thirds of the time indicated on the package directions. Drain well and transfer to a bowl.

3. Meanwhile, in a medium nonstick saucepan, combine 3 cups water, ¾ teaspoon salt, and the cumin and paprika. Bring to a boil and add the rutabaga. Cook for 3 minutes, or until just soft. Remove from the heat and stir in the pork. Reserving the broth, strain out the rutabaga and pork and add to the pasta. Measure out 2 cups of the broth.

4. Wipe the saucepan and heat the oil over medium-high heat. Add the bell pepper and sprinkle with a pinch of salt. Cook for 1 minute. Stir in the flour until well incorporated. Slowly whisk in the milk and broth and bring to a simmer, then cook for 1 minute. Off the heat, stir in 3 tablespoons of the Parmesan and ¼ teaspoon black pepper.

5. Add the sauce to the bowl with the rutabaga and pork and toss to combine. Transfer the mixture to the baking dish. Sprinkle the remaining 5 tablespoons Parmesan evenly over the top and grind on a little black pepper.

6. Bake for 25 to 30 minutes, or until the top is browned and the filling is lightly bubbling. Let stand for 10 minutes before serving.

Per serving: 379 calories • 24g protein • 12g fat (3.5g saturated) • 3.5g fiber • 44g carbohydrate • 523mg sodium • 38mg magnesium

Thai Curry Rice Bowl

Hands-On Time: 15 minutes | **Total Time:** 55 minutes | **Makes:** 4 servings

A typical Thai curry is made with coconut milk and flavored with fresh herbs—usually some combination of basil, mint, and cilantro. This, also includes turmeric and ginger for their belly-friendly properties. To save time, make the rice ahead of time and freeze for up to 3 months. To reheat, place the rice in a covered microwaveable bowl with 2 tablespoons of water and cook for 3 minutes on 50% power.

- ⅔ cup long-grain brown rice
- 2 cups water
- 2 teaspoons chia seeds
- 2 teaspoons sesame seeds (roasted, if available)
- ⅛ teaspoon plus ½ teaspoon salt
- 1 tablespoon plus 1 teaspoon extra-virgin olive oil
- 1 tablespoon grated fresh ginger
- 1 teaspoon turmeric
- 1 medium eggplant (1 pound), cut into ¾-inch chunks
- 1¼ pounds boneless, skinless chicken breast, cut into ¾-inch chunks
- ¾ cup light coconut milk
- ⅓ cup chopped fresh basil
- ⅓ cup chopped fresh cilantro, mint, or a combination

BELLY BUDDIES: Brown rice, chia seeds, sesame seeds, olive oil, ginger, turmeric, eggplant, chicken breast, coconut milk

1. In a small saucepan, combine the rice, 1½ cups of the water, the chia seeds, sesame seeds, and ⅛ teaspoon of the salt. Bring to a boil, then reduce to a simmer, cover, and cook for 40 minutes. Remove from the heat and let stand, covered, for 10 minutes. Fluff with a fork and cover to keep warm.

2. Meanwhile, in a nonstick Dutch oven, heat the oil over medium-high heat. Add the ginger and turmeric and stir for 30 seconds, or until fragrant. Add the eggplant, sprinkle with ½ teaspoon salt, and toss to coat. Add the remaining ½ cup water, cover, and simmer for 5 minutes, or until the eggplant is just softening.

3. Add the chicken and toss to combine. Add the coconut milk and bring to a boil. Reduce to a simmer, cover, and cook for 5 minutes, or until the chicken is cooked through and the eggplant is fully tender. Stir in the fresh herbs.

4. Serve the eggplant-chicken mixture over the rice.

Per serving: 400 calories • 35g protein • 14g fat (4.5g saturated) • 7g fiber • 33g carbohydrate • 547mg sodium • 117mg magnesium

If you have gluten issues: Choose a gluten-free brand of chia seeds.

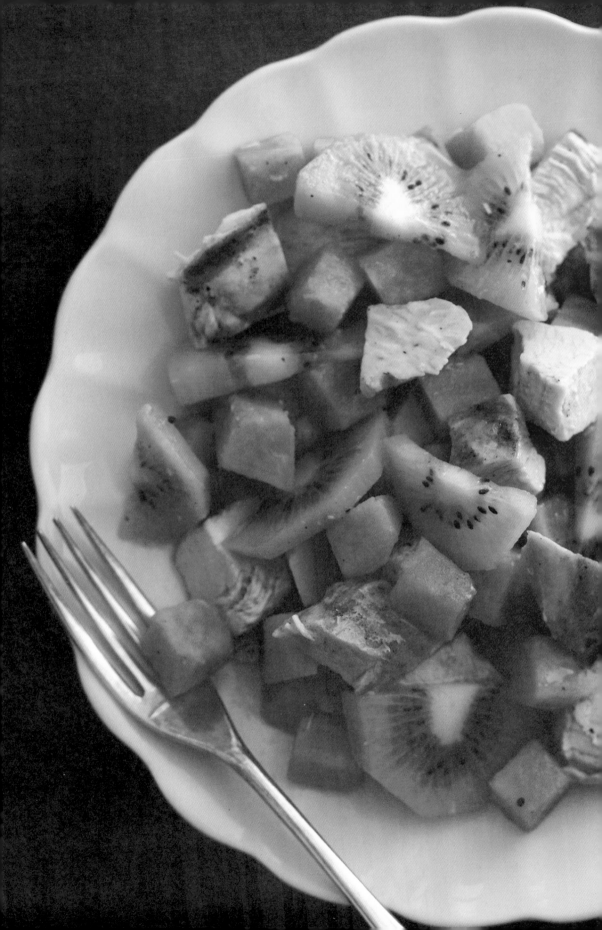

Grilled Chicken, Sweet Potato, and Kiwi Salad

Hands-On Time: 25 minutes | **Total Time:** 25 minutes | **Makes:** 4 (1¾-cup) servings

When making this ahead, do not add the kiwi until just before serving. Kiwis have enzymes that will make the chicken mushy. If you are planning to have leftovers, store the kiwi separately and add it only when you're ready to eat.

1¼ pounds boneless, skinless chicken breasts

2 teaspoons sesame oil

1 pound sweet potatoes, peeled and cut into ½-inch cubes (about 3 medium potatoes)

2 tablespoons fresh lime juice

1 tablespoon plus 1 teaspoon extra-virgin olive oil

½ teaspoon salt

3 kiwis, peeled and cut into ½-inch cubes

BELLY BUDDIES: Chicken breast, sesame oil, olive oil, kiwi

1. In a shallow bowl, toss the chicken with the sesame oil.

2. Heat a grill pan over medium-high heat. Add the chicken and cook for 5 minutes without turning. Flip and cook for 5 to 7 minutes, or until cooked through but still juicy. Transfer to a cutting board and let sit for 10 minutes before cutting into ½-inch cubes.

3. In a vegetable steamer, cook the sweet potatoes for 5 minutes, or until tender.

4. In a small bowl, whisk together the lime juice, olive oil, and salt.

5. In a large bowl, toss together the chicken, sweet potatoes, kiwi, and dressing.

Per serving: 322 calories • 32g protein • 11g fat (2g saturated) • 4g fiber • 24g carbohydrate • 481mg sodium • 62mg magnesium

Test Team Fave!

"One night I was cutting some kiwi for myself when my 2-year-old daughter Trista pointed to it and said, 'Can I have some of you that?' I handed her some and told her to try it. She said, 'I can't. I 'fraid.' My husband chimed in and said, 'Afraid of what? Mommy is eating it.' She replied, 'Daddy eat it.'

"As soon as John put his piece in his mouth, she ate hers. 'Mmmmm! That's good! More?'

"A day or two later was the sweet potato and kiwi salad. I cut up all of the kiwi and was waiting on the sweet potatoes and chicken when a small hand emerged from under the island and reached up. 'Riwi?' Trista ate so much of the 'riwi' that I had to cut up another one.

"I love that I'm introducing my daughter to healthy foods and that she likes them!" —TONYA CARKEET

Crunchy Chicken Couscous

Hands-On Time: 20 minutes | **Total Time:** 30 minutes | **Makes:** 4 (1¾-cup) servings

"Shredding" carrots with a vegetable peeler is fast and easy and produces long ribbons that cook quickly. To do it, use the same motions as when you're peeling the carrot. Turmeric soothes your aggravated digestive tract and also infuses food with an earthy-mustard flavor. You'll find roasted brown rice couscous in the gluten-free section of most grocery stores. If you like, all the ingredients can be prepped early in the day and refrigerated separately.

BELLY BUDDIES:
Olive oil, carrot, zucchini, brown rice, turmeric, chicken breast, tomatoes, peanuts

- 1 tablespoon extra-virgin olive oil
- 1 medium carrot, shredded with a vegetable peeler
- 1 zucchini (6 ounces), quartered lengthwise and cut crosswise into ½-inch-thick pieces
- ½ cup roasted brown rice couscous
- ½ teaspoon salt
- ½ teaspoon ground coriander
- ½ teaspoon turmeric
- 1⅓ cups water
- 1 pound boneless, skinless chicken breasts, cut into 1-inch chunks
- 2 plum tomatoes, diced
- ½ cup chopped fresh cilantro
- 2 tablespoons coarsely chopped unsalted peanuts

1. In a medium saucepan, heat the oil over medium heat. Add the carrot and zucchini and cook, stirring frequently, for 3 minutes, or until the carrot is wilted and the zucchini is crisp-tender.

2. Add the couscous, salt, coriander, turmeric, and water and bring to a boil. Reduce to a simmer, add the chicken and tomatoes, cover, and simmer for 7 to 8 minutes, or until the couscous is tender and the chicken is cooked through.

3. Stir in the cilantro and peanuts. Serve hot.

Per serving: 283 calories • 28g protein • 9.5g fat (1.5g saturated) • 3g fiber • 23g carbohydrate • 438mg sodium • 51mg magnesium

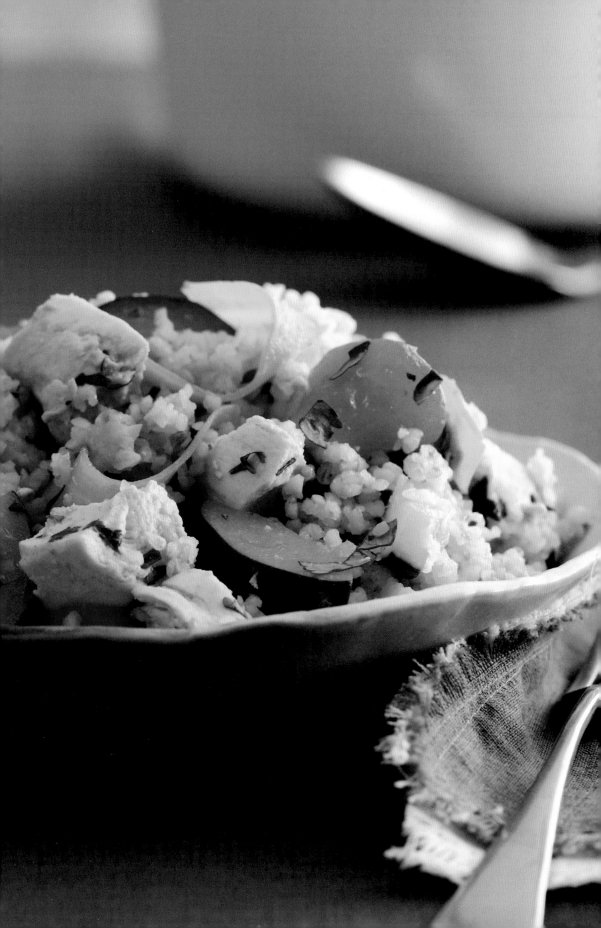

Lemony Salmon, Potato, and Dill Bake

Hands-On Time: 20 minutes | **Total Time:** 55 minutes | **Makes:** 4 servings

You can purchase shredded cabbage packed in bags in the produce department. Or, if you'd like, you can swap in kale for the cabbage, using the same amount and cooking it in the same way. Salmon, one of the best omega-3 fat sources on earth, delivers a big dose of calm to your sensitive gut.

BELLY BUDDIES:
Potatoes, green cabbage, lemon, olive oil, salmon

- 1 pound red potatoes, cut into ½-inch-thick slices
- 1 pound green cabbage, shredded (about 6 cups)
- 1 lemon, halved, seeded, and cut into ½-inch chunks
- ½ cup sliced scallion greens
- ½ cup chopped fresh dill
- ½ cup water
- ½ teaspoon salt
- 2 teaspoons extra-virgin olive oil
- 4 skinless salmon fillets (about 5 ounces each)

1. Preheat the oven to 450°F. In a large saucepan of boiling water, cook the potatoes for 5 minutes to blanch. Drain well.

2. In a 9 x 13-inch baking dish, combine the potatoes, cabbage, lemon, scallion greens, dill, water, salt, and oil and toss well to combine. Cover with foil and bake for 20 minutes, or until the cabbage is crisp-tender.

3. Uncover and place the salmon on top of the cabbage mixture. Bake for 7 to 10 minutes, or until the salmon is slightly firm, does not flake, and is cooked to medium. Serve the salmon with the vegetables.

Per serving: 435 calories • 33g protein • 22g fat (4.5g saturated) • 6g fiber • 28g carbohydrate • 423mg sodium • 70mg magnesium

Test Team Fave!

"Could this Lemony Salmon, Potato, and Dill Bake possibly be the best meal I've ever had? OMG!" —ADRIENNE FARR

"Caprese" Pasta Salad

Hands-On Time: 10 minutes | **Total Time:** 40 minutes | **Makes:** 4 servings

Eight cubes of baked tofu has 93 calories and 8 grams of protein, making it a great source of lean protein. Using it instead of mozzarella in this salad reduces the amount of tummy-troubling lactose, while adding pasta (gluten-free to reduce your intake of troublesome gassy carbs found in wheat-rich foods) makes it a hearty stand-alone meal.

You can bake the tofu for this up to 5 days ahead. In fact, the baked tofu on its own makes a perfectly nice snack. (If you want to make some extra for that purpose, you might want to add a little spice to the tofu before you bake it: Try cumin or onion- and garlic-free curry or chili powder.)

1 package (14 ounces) extra-firm tofu, drained

2 teaspoons coconut oil, melted

1 teaspoon coarse (kosher) salt

4 ounces gluten-free quinoa elbow macaroni

1 tablespoon plus 1 teaspoon balsamic vinegar

1 tablespoon extra-virgin olive oil

¼ teaspoon black pepper

3 plum tomatoes, cut into smallish chunks

⅓ cup torn fresh basil

5 cups packed baby spinach (5 ounces)

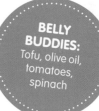

BELLY BUDDIES: Tofu, olive oil, tomatoes, spinach

1. Preheat the oven to 400°F. Line a baking sheet with parchment paper.

2. Halve the block of tofu horizontally, then cut each slab of tofu into 20 cubes (for a total of 40). In a large bowl, toss the tofu with the coconut oil. Spread on the baking sheet and roast for 25 to 30 minutes, or until firm and beginning to brown. Remove from the oven, return to the same bowl, sprinkle with ½ teaspoon of the salt, toss to coat, and let cool to room temperature.

3. Meanwhile, cook the pasta according to package directions using the remaining ½ teaspoon salt. Drain, rinse under cool water, and drain well.

4. In a small bowl or screw-top jar, mix together the vinegar, olive oil, and pepper.

5. Add the pasta, tomatoes, basil, and 2 teaspoons of the vinaigrette to the tofu and toss well. In a separate bowl, toss the spinach with the remaining vinaigrette.

6. To serve, mound the tofu-tomato mixture on a bed of the spinach.

Per serving: 277 calories • 13g protein • 11g fat (3g saturated) • 5.5g fiber • 32g carbohydrate • 546mg sodium • 8mg magnesium

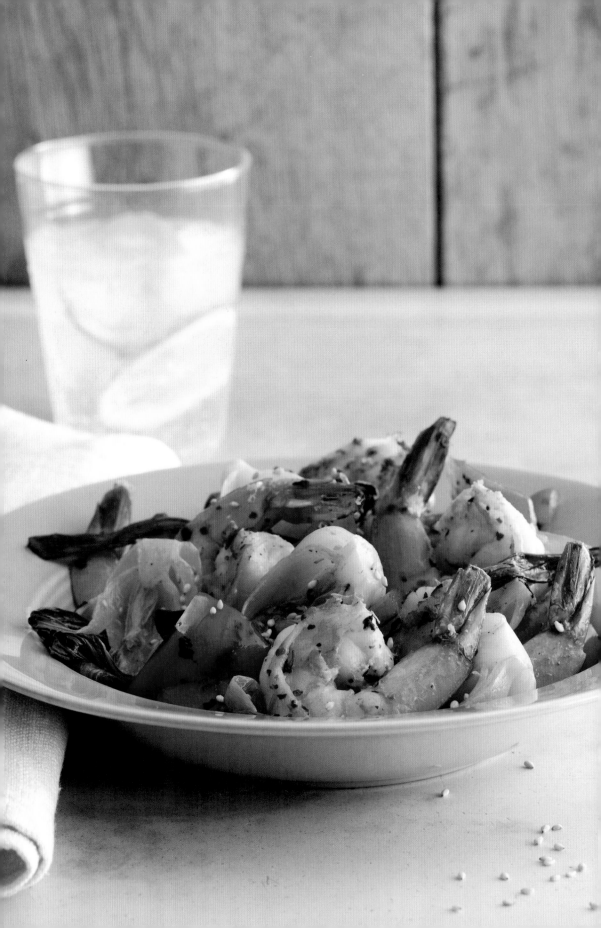

Herb-Roasted Shrimp

Hands-On Time: 15 minutes | **Total Time:** 35 minutes | **Makes:** 4 servings

The combo of bell peppers, bok choy, scallion greens, and shrimp is reminiscent of an Asian stir-fry. But instead of stirring in a wok, we've chosen to roast the vegetables and shrimp together. It's easier and equally delicious. If you can't find baby bok choy, swap in regular—simply cut it into 2-inch chunks. If you've got leftovers, this makes a great cold lunch. Low in gas-producing FODMAPs, it will pacify and nourish your digestive system.

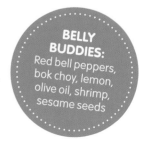

BELLY BUDDIES: Red bell peppers, bok choy, lemon, olive oil, shrimp, sesame seeds

- 2 red bell peppers, cut into large squares
- ¾ pound baby bok choy, halved lengthwise
- 1½ cups 2-inch lengths scallion greens
- 1 tablespoon plus 1 teaspoon fresh lemon juice
- ¼ teaspoon salt
- 4 teaspoons extra-virgin olive oil
- 1 pound (about 24) peeled and deveined large shrimp
- 1 teaspoon dried basil
- ½ teaspoon grated lemon zest
- 2 teaspoons sesame seeds

1. Preheat the oven to 400°F.

2. In a 9 x 13-inch baking dish, toss together the bell peppers, bok choy, scallion greens, lemon juice, salt, and 2 teaspoons of the oil.

3. In a small bowl, toss together the shrimp, basil, lemon zest, and remaining 2 teaspoons oil.

4. Scatter the shrimp over the vegetables and roast for 20 minutes, or until the shrimp are just cooked through. Serve with the sesame seeds sprinkled on top.

Per serving: 186 calories • 24g protein • 7.5g fat (1g saturated) • 2.5g fiber • 7g carbohydrate • 441mg sodium • 36mg magnesium

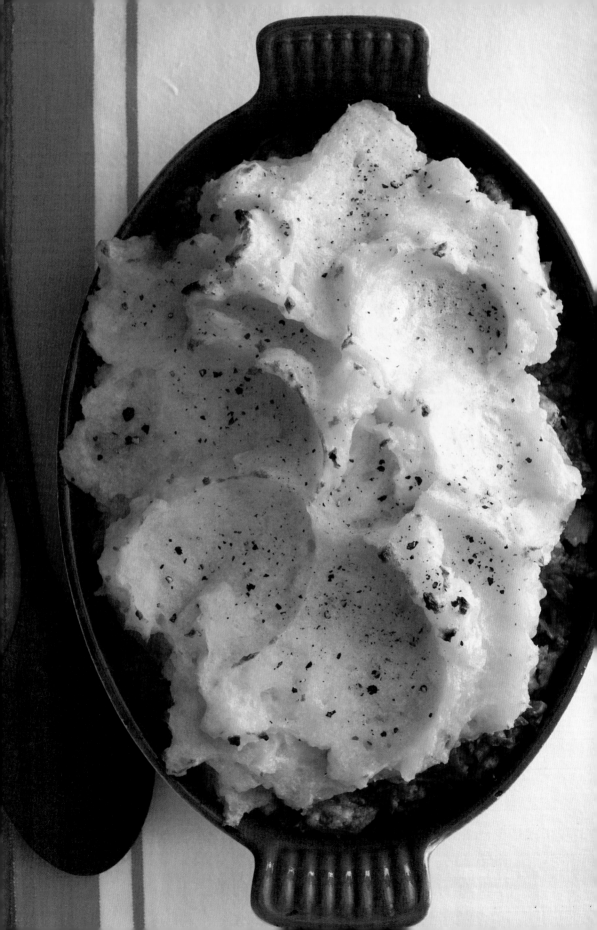

Vegetarian Shepherd's Pie

Hands-On Time: 30 minutes | **Total Time:** 1 hour 20 minutes |
Makes: 6 servings

You can make the filling for the shepherd's pie a day ahead and refrigerate, but let it come back to room temperature before putting together the pie. Make the potato-parsnip topping just before assembling the pie, which should be done no more than an hour before baking. Tofu provides a nice dose of vegetarian protein that is devoid of the gas-producing fibers found in other traditional "veggie" protein sources such as kidney beans and many other legumes.

Filling:

- 2 carrots, peeled and cut into chunks
- ¼ small head green cabbage, cut into large chunks
- 1 tablespoon plus 1 teaspoon extra-virgin olive oil
- ½ teaspoon crumbled dried rosemary
- ½ teaspoon salt
- 1 container (14 ounces) extra-firm tofu, drained
- ⅓ cup finely chopped walnuts

- 1¼ cups canned no-salt-added crushed tomatoes
- 2 teaspoons Worcestershire sauce

Olive oil spray

Topping:

- 1 teaspoon turmeric
- 1 teaspoon salt
- 10 ounces parsnips, peeled and thinly sliced
- 10 ounces russet (baking) potato, thinly sliced
- ¾ cup shredded reduced-fat cheddar cheese (3 ounces)

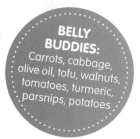

BELLY BUDDIES: Carrots, cabbage, olive oil, tofu, walnuts, tomatoes, turmeric, parsnips, potatoes

1. To make the filling: In a food processor, finely chop the carrots until they are the texture of cooked ground meat. Transfer to a bowl. Add the cabbage to the processor (no need to clean) and process the same way.

2. In a large nonstick skillet, heat the oil over medium heat. Add the carrots, cabbage, rosemary, and ¼ teaspoon of the salt and cook, stirring often, for 5 to 7 minutes, or until the cabbage and carrots are beginning to soften. Crumble in the tofu and break it up with a fork into fine crumbles. Add the nuts, tomatoes, Worcestershire sauce, and remaining ¼ teaspoon salt and cook for 5 minutes to blend the flavors and cook off some of the liquid.

3. Preheat the oven to 375°F. Lightly coat a 9-inch square baking pan with olive oil spray.

(continued on page 200)

(continued from page 199)

Vegetarian Shepherd's Pie

4. To make the topping: Bring a medium pot of water to a boil. Add the turmeric, salt, parsnips, and potato and cook for 5 to 7 minutes, or until very tender. Reserving the cooking liquid, drain well and return to the pot. Mash well using some of the reserved cooking water to make a spreadable mixture. Stir in the cheese to combine.

5. Pour the filling in the baking pan and spread the topping over it. Place in the oven and bake for 30 to 35 minutes, or until the top is lightly browned. Let stand for 10 minutes before serving.

Per serving: 294 calories • 14g protein • 15g fat (3.5g saturated) • 6.5g fiber • 27g carbohydrate • 373mg sodium • 58mg magnesium

If you have gluten issues: Choose a gluten-free brand of Worcestershire sauce.

Test Team Fave!

"The Vegetarian Shepherd's Pie? Wow. Oh wow. Love! It's great to have some nice, cold-weather, comfort-food-style recipes." —TONYA CARKEET

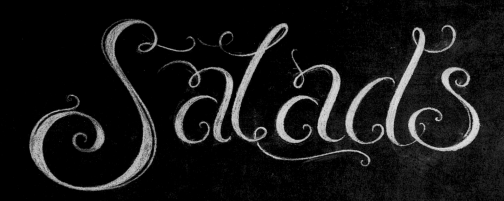

Salads

CARB-LIGHT, HIGH-FIBER GREENS TAKE THE SPOTLIGHT

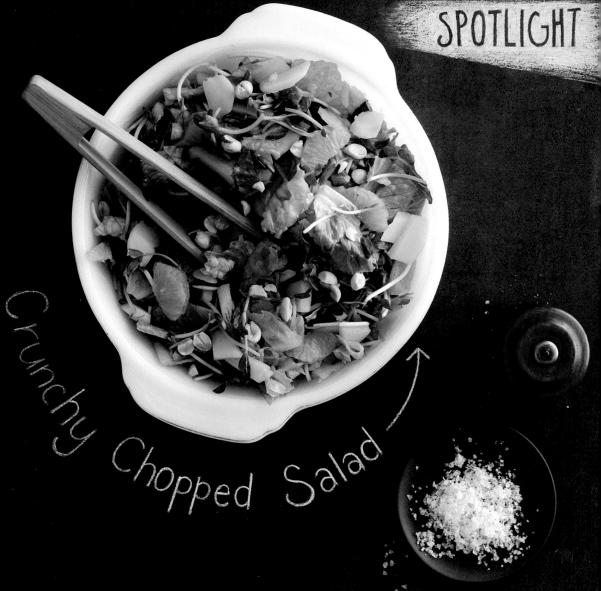

Crunchy Chopped Salad

Crunchy Chopped Salad

Hands-On Time: 15 minutes | **Total Time:** 15 minutes | **Makes:** 4 (2-cup) servings

To turn this side salad into a main course, grill up some shrimp or chicken breasts (about 6 ounces per person) and serve on top of the salad. Coat the chicken or shrimp with a little soy sauce and extra-virgin olive oil (or Roasted Garlic Oil, page 211) before grilling.

BELLY BUDDIES: Tangerines, olive oil, lettuce, water chestnuts, peanuts

2   large tangerines

1   tablespoon extra-virgin olive oil

2   teaspoons reduced-sodium soy sauce

¼   teaspoon salt

Pinch of cayenne pepper

4   cups chopped romaine lettuce

4   cups fresh sunflower sprouts (or other largish fresh sprout, such as pea shoots), coarsely chopped

1   can (8 ounces) sliced water chestnuts, diced

8   teaspoons chopped unsalted peanuts

1. Halve one of the tangerines and squeeze the juice into a small bowl. Whisk in the oil, soy sauce, salt, and cayenne.

2. Peel the remaining tangerine, divide into sections, and cut into small pieces, discarding the seeds as you do.

3. In a large bowl, toss together the romaine, sprouts, water chestnuts, and tangerines. Add half the tangerine vinaigrette and toss again.

4. Divide the salad among 4 salad plates and drizzle the remaining dressing over the salads. Top each serving with 2 teaspoons of the peanuts.

Per serving: 121 calories • 4g protein • 6.5g fat (1g saturated) • 4g fiber • 14g carbohydrate • 252mg sodium • 28mg magnesium

If you have gluten issues: Choose a gluten-free brand of soy sauce.

Butter Lettuce with Scallion-Ginger Vinaigrette

Hands-On Time: 10 minutes | **Total Time:** 20 minutes | **Makes:** 4 (2-cup) servings

Even though raw scallion whites can spell digestive problems for people, you can still take advantage of their wonderful flavor by using them to infuse oil. Since the offending substances in scallions are not oil soluble, the oil will taste like scallions but won't upset your tummy. (If you have leftover scallion whites from any of the other recipes in this book, use them here.) As an added bonus, the scallion oil here also contains ginger, which soothes and calms while infusing food with a wonderful flavor.

- 3 scallions, chopped, white and greens kept separate
- ½ inch fresh ginger, very thinly sliced (no need to peel)
- 2 tablespoons almond oil or extra-virgin olive oil
- 1 tablespoon plus 1 teaspoon unseasoned rice vinegar
- ⅛ teaspoon salt
- ⅛ teaspoon black pepper
- 1 large or 2 small heads Boston, Bibb, or butter lettuce, torn into leaves (8 to 10 cups)
- 2 tablespoons sliced almonds (toasted, if desired)

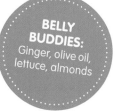

BELLY BUDDIES:
Ginger, olive oil, lettuce, almonds

1. In a small saucepan, combine the scallion whites, all but 2 tablespoons of the greens (which are set aside), the ginger, and oil. Heat over low heat, stirring, for 5 minutes, or until the scallions are softened and the oil is quite fragrant. Remove from the heat and set aside to steep and cool to room temperature.

2. Strain the scallion-ginger oil into a small bowl, pressing on the solids to get as much oil as possible (discard the solids). Whisk in the vinegar, salt, and pepper.

3. In a large salad bowl, add the lettuce and toss with the vinaigrette. Divide among 4 salad plates and sprinkle with the reserved scallion greens and sliced almonds.

Per serving: 72 calories • 1g protein • 7g fat (0.5g saturated) • 1g fiber • 2g carbohydrate • 75mg sodium • 13mg magnesium

Grape and Walnut Waldorf Salad

Hands-On Time: 25 minutes | **Total Time:** 25 minutes | **Makes:** 4 servings

Subtract the apples (which are Belly Bullies) from a classic Waldorf salad and you still wind up with a refreshing dish. A mildly sweet dressing of Greek yogurt, mayo, and maple syrup dresses up greens, celery, grapes, and nuts. Greek yogurt has less lactose than traditional yogurt and a dose of probiotics (healthy bacteria), making this dressing belly friendly. Serve the salad with Herb-Roasted Shrimp (page 197) or Vegetarian Shepherd's Pie (page 199).

BELLY BUDDIES: Greek yogurt, maple syrup, lemon, grapes, walnuts, lettuce

- ⅔ cup nonfat plain Greek yogurt
- 2 tablespoons olive oil mayonnaise
- 1 tablespoon pure maple syrup
- 1 tablespoon fresh lemon juice
- 2 tablespoons chopped fresh parsley
- ¼ teaspoon salt
- 3 ribs celery, thinly sliced
- 1 cup seedless red grapes (about 40), halved
- ⅓ cup walnuts or pecans, coarsely chopped
- 1 small head Boston lettuce, torn into large pieces

In a medium bowl, whisk together the yogurt, mayonnaise, maple syrup, lemon juice, parsley, and salt. Fold in the celery, grapes, and walnuts. Divide the lettuce among 4 plates and top each with the salad mixture.

Per serving: 153 calories • 6g protein • 7.5g fat (1g saturated) • 2g fiber • 17g carbohydrate • 253mg sodium • 27mg magnesium

If you have gluten issues: Choose gluten-free brands of Greek yogurt.

Tomato Lime Quinoa Salad

Hands-On Time: 15 minutes | **Total Time:** 35 minutes | **Makes:** 8 (½-cup) servings

Quinoa is a versatile, carb-light grain that cooks quickly and pairs well with fresh tomatoes and lime. Refrigerate any leftovers; they'll keep for up to 4 days. This can be served warm or cool, as a hearty side dish or as a stand-alone salad.

1 cup quinoa, soaked for about 15 minutes, drained, and rinsed

2 limes, juiced

3 scallion greens, cut in thin rounds

2 medium tomatoes, seeded and cut into small chunks

1 tablespoon extra-virgin olive oil

¾ teaspoon cumin

Pinch of salt

Black pepper

2 tablespoons chopped fresh dill or cilantro

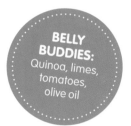

BELLY BUDDIES: Quinoa, limes, tomatoes, olive oil

1. Cook the quinoa according to package directions and let cool. Place in a medium bowl.

2. Add the lime juice (to taste), scallions, tomatoes, oil, cumin (to taste), and salt to the quinoa and stir together.

3. Season to taste with pepper. Garnish with the dill.

Per serving: 104 calories • 3g protein • 3g fat (0g saturated) • 1.5g fiber • 17g carbohydrate • 25mg sodium • 5mg magnesium

Kale Caesar Salad

Hands-On Time: 15 minutes | **Total Time:** 25 minutes | **Makes:** 4 servings

There are several varieties of kale on the market. Curly kale, pictured here, is the most common. Tuscan kale (also called lacinato, dinosaur, or black kale) has blue-green leaves and a sweeter flavor than curly. Russian kale has sweet reddish leaves. Any of the varieties would work here. To make this into a main-dish salad, top with grilled chicken breast or pork tenderloin (about 5 ounces per person).

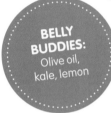

BELLY BUDDIES:
Olive oil, kale, lemon

3 (6-inch) corn tortillas

2 teaspoons extra-virgin olive oil

1 pound kale

2 tablespoons olive oil mayonnaise

2 tablespoons fresh lemon juice

2 anchovy fillets, mashed (1 teaspoon)

⅓ cup grated Parmesan cheese

1. Preheat the oven to 375°F.

2. Place the tortillas on a baking sheet and brush one side with the oil. Bake for 10 minutes, or until the tortillas are crisp and browned around the edges. Cool on the baking sheet, then break into large pieces.

3. Grab the stem end of each kale leaf and, pushing upward, strip the leaves off the stalks. Tear each leaf into bite-size pieces (discard the stalks).

4. Fill a Dutch oven or large saucepan with water to come up about 3 inches. Bring the water to a boil, add the kale, and cover the

pan. Cook for 5 minutes, or until the kale is tender but not mushy. Drain, rinse under cold water to stop the cooking, then drain well and pat dry.

5. Meanwhile, in a large bowl, whisk together the mayonnaise, lemon juice, and anchovies until well combined. Whisk in the cheese.

6. Add the kale to the bowl with the dressing and toss to coat. Divide among 4 plates and scatter the tortilla chips over the top.

Per serving: 151 calories • 6g protein • 7g fat (2g saturated) • 2.5g fiber • 17g carbohydrate • 264mg sodium • 39mg magnesium

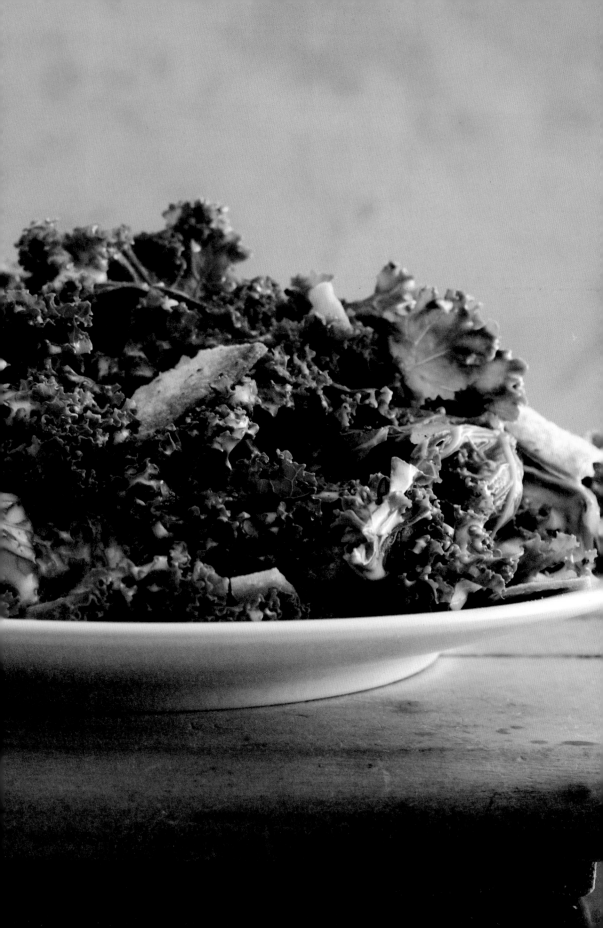

Mustard-y Dressing

Hands-On Time: 5 minutes | **Total Time:** 5 minutes | **Makes:** ½ cup

Spice up grilled chickien or fish with this teriffic tangy dressing.

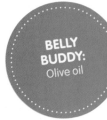

BELLY BUDDY: Olive oil

- 2 tablespoons red wine vinegar
- 1 tablespoon chopped chives
- ¼ teaspoon sea salt
- 2 teaspoons Dijon mustard
- ⅓ cup extra-virgin olive oil

1. In a small bowl, mix the vinegar, chives, and salt and let sit for a minute to infuse flavor.

2. In another small bowl, add the mustard to the oil and whisk to blend. Add to the vinegar mixture and mix well.

Per teaspoon: 27 calories • 0g protein • 3g fat (0.5g saturated) • 0g fiber • 0g carbohydrate • 34mg sodium • 0mg magnesium

If you have gluten issues: Choose a gluten-free brand of mustard.

Asian Sesame Dressing

Hands-On Time: 5 minutes | **Total Time:** 5 minutes | **Makes:** ¾ cup

Use this onion- and garlic-free dressing on any green salad. Store in the refrigerator for up to a week.

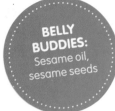

BELLY BUDDIES: Sesame oil, sesame seeds

- ⅓ cup peanut oil
- 2 tablespoons sesame oil
- 3 tablespoons rice vinegar
- 2 tablespoons reduced-sodium soy sauce
- 2 teaspoons toasted sesame seeds
- ¼ cup thinly sliced scallion greens

In a medium bowl, combine the oils, vinegar, soy sauce, sesame seeds, and scallion greens. Whisk to blend.

Per teaspoon: 26 calories • 0g protein • 3g fat (0.5g saturated) • 0g fiber • 0g carbohydrate • 39mg sodium • 0mg magnesium

If you have gluten issues: Choose a gluten-free brand of soy sauce.

◄SIDES►

SIMPLY GOOD FOR YOUR GUT

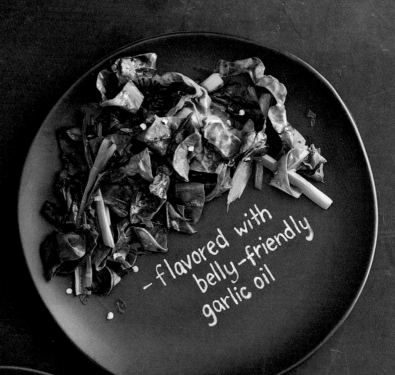

—flavored with belly-friendly garlic oil

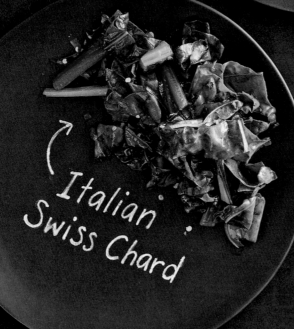

Italian Swiss Chard

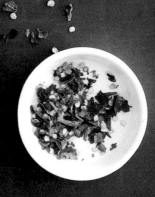

Italian Swiss Chard

Hands-On Time: 15 minutes | **Total Time:** 15 minutes | **Makes:** 4 (½-cup) servings

Swiss chard—a much underrated vegetable—comes in a rainbow of colors. The leaves stay the same (green), but the stems and the veins in the leaves can be white, red, or yellow. In fact, some markets even sell what they call "rainbow chard," which is all three chard colors bundled together. Leftovers of the chard make a nice salad; just add a little lemon juice or vinegar to taste.

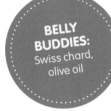

BELLY BUDDIES: Swiss chard, olive oil

- 1 bunch Swiss chard (1 pound)
- 1 tablespoon Roasted Garlic Oil (recipe follows)
- ½ teaspoon dried oregano
- ¼ teaspoon red-pepper flakes (optional)
- ¼ teaspoon salt

1. Cut the stems and wide portions of the center ribs away from the chard leaves. Trim the ends of the stems and cut the stems crosswise into ½-inch pieces. Halve the leaves lengthwise and cut crosswise into ½-inch shreds. Wash the chard well in a large bowl of water (letting the sand fall to the bottom). Drain the leaves, but leave them a bit wet.

2. In a large skillet, heat the oil, oregano, pepper flakes (if using), and salt over medium-high heat. Add the chard stems and cook for 2 minutes.

3. Add all of the chard leaves at once, cover the skillet, and cook for 1 minute. Uncover, stir the chard to coat with the oil and spices, then re-cover and cook for 1 minute, or until wilted and tender.

Per serving: 52 calories • 2g protein • 3.5g fat (0.5g saturated) • 2g fiber • 4g carbohydrate • 387mg sodium • 92mg magnesium

Roasted Garlic Oil

When olive oil is refrigerated, it will get cloudy or even solidify. This is natural. Just let it come back to room temperature. Or, if you're in a rush, run the oil container under hot running water, which will immediately reliquefy the oil. Garlic is a Belly Bully, but this garlic-infused oil just takes the flavor of the garlic and keeps the bullies out.

¾ cup extra-virgin olive oil

12 cloves garlic, peeled and thickly sliced

1. Preheat the oven to 325°F.

2. Combine the oil and garlic in a very small baking dish (a mini loaf pan or a 10-ounce ramekin would work). The garlic should be submerged. Cover tightly with foil and place on a baking sheet. Bake for 35 to 45 minutes, or until the garlic is just beginning to turn color. Check often toward the end because you don't want the garlic to get too dark.

3. Let the garlic cool in the oil. Strain out and discard the garlic. Store the oil in the fridge.

Creamed Spinach

Hands-On Time: 10 minutes | **Total Time:** 20 minutes | **Makes:** 4 (⅔-cup) servings

My daughters like spinach, especially when I combine it with creamy ingredients like milk and cream cheese. The spinach is topped with the heroes of the seed world, chia seeds. They are high in omega-3s, help reduce food cravings, and may help lower your blood pressure.

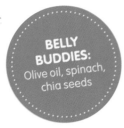

BELLY BUDDIES: Olive oil, spinach, chia seeds

2 teaspoons extra-virgin olive oil

1 bag (16 ounces) frozen chopped spinach, thawed and squeezed dry

½ teaspoon dried oregano or thyme

½ teaspoon salt

1 cup lactose-free 1% milk

4 tablespoons (2 ounces) ⅓-less-fat cream cheese

2 teaspoons chia seeds

1. In a large saucepan, heat the oil over medium-low heat. Add the spinach, oregano, and salt and cook, stirring occasionally, for 5 minutes, or until the spinach is tender.

2. Add the milk and cream cheese and cook, stirring occasionally, for 10 minutes, or until thick and creamy.

3. Serve hot, sprinkled with the chia seeds.

Per serving: 123 calories • 8g protein • 7.5g fat (2.5g saturated) • 4g fiber • 9g carbohydrate • 453mg sodium • 101mg magnesium

If you have gluten issues: Choose a gluten-free brand of chia seeds.

Parmesan-Crumbed Kale

Hands-On Time: 10 minutes | **Total Time:** 30 minutes | **Makes:** 4 (1¼-cup) servings

While any type of kale can be used in this recipe, Tuscan kale (also called laci-nato, dinosaur, or black kale) is called for because it's easier to strip the long leaves off the stems. Kale is rich in flavonoids, key anti-inflammation busters that help calm and flatten the belly. Ground corn tortillas along with Parme-san cheese and a little olive oil make a nice, crisp topping that can be used on other vegetables, such as broiled tomato slices or sautéed green beans.

1 bunch Tuscan kale (12 ounces)
2 (6-inch) corn tortillas
½ cup grated Parmesan cheese

¼ teaspoon salt
⅛ teaspoon cayenne pepper
3 teaspoons Roasted Garlic Oil (page 211)

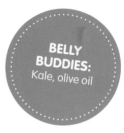

BELLY BUDDIES:
Kale, olive oil

1. Preheat the oven to 375°F.

2. Grab the stem end of each kale leaf and, pushing upward, strip the leaves off the stems. Tear the leaves into bite-size pieces.

3. Fill a Dutch oven or large saucepan with water to come up about 3 inches. Bring the water to a boil, add the kale, and cover the pan. Cook for 5 minutes, or until the kale is tender but not mushy. Drain, rinse under cold water to stop the cooking, then drain well.

4. Place the tortillas in a food processor and pulse until finely ground. Add the Parmesan, salt, cayenne, and 1 teaspoon of the oil and pulse to combine.

5. Place the kale in a 9 x 9-inch baking dish, sprinkle with the remaining 2 teaspoons oil, and toss well. Sprinkle the cheese mixture over the kale. Bake for 15 minutes, or until the topping is lightly browned and crisp and the kale is piping hot.

Per serving: 128 calories • 6g protein • 7g fat (2.5g saturated) • 1.5g fiber • 12g carbohy-drate • 322mg sodium • 30mg magnesium

Green Beans Amandine

Hands-On Time: 15 minutes | Total Time: 25 minutes | **Makes:** 4 (1¼-cup) servings

A small amount of lemon zest and juice brighten up this simple dish. If you can, choose thin green beans (they'll be tastier) and try to get beans that are all about the same size, so they'll cook in the same amount of time. If you'd like to spice this dish up a bit, add a tablespoon of peeled and minced fresh ginger when steaming the beans and bell pepper.

BELLY BUDDIES: Olive oil, red bell pepper, green beans, lemon, almonds

- 1 tablespoon extra-virgin olive oil
- 1 red bell pepper, cut into thin strips
- 1 pound green beans, trimmed
- ½ teaspoon salt
- ¼ teaspoon black pepper
- ½ cup water
- 1 teaspoon grated lemon zest
- 1 tablespoon fresh lemon juice
- ¼ cup slivered almonds

1. In a large skillet, heat the oil over medium-low heat. Add the bell pepper and green beans and stir to coat. Add the salt, black pepper, and water and bring to a boil. Reduce the heat to a simmer and cook for 7 to 10 minutes, or until the green beans are tender.

2. Add the lemon zest, lemon juice, and almonds and toss to combine. Serve hot, at room temperature, or chilled.

Per serving: 115 calories • 4g protein • 7g fat (1g saturated) • 4.5g fiber • 12g carbohydrate • 299mg sodium • 51mg magnesium

Summer Squash Gratin

Hands-On Time: 20 minutes | **Total Time:** 35 minutes | **Makes:** 6 (1¼-cup) servings

In August, backyard gardens are overflowing with summer squash and zucchini, but don't be tempted to use the superlarge ones; they're seedy and not particularly flavorful (leave them for the birds). Smaller are better—sweeter, firmer, and less seedy—and if you can find golden zucchini, go for them as they're even tastier.

1 tablespoon plus 1 teaspoon extra-virgin olive oil

2 yellow summer squash (about 6 ounces each), thinly sliced

2 zucchini (about 6 ounces each), thinly sliced

½ teaspoon salt

¾ cup lactose-free 1% milk

½ cup grated Parmesan cheese

⅓ cup almond flour

2 tablespoons oat bran

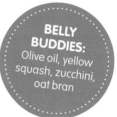

BELLY BUDDIES: Olive oil, yellow squash, zucchini, oat bran

1. Preheat the oven to 450°F.

2. In a large nonstick skillet, heat the oil over medium heat. Add the yellow squash, zucchini, and salt. Cover and cook, stirring occasionally, for 7 minutes, or until the squash is tender.

3. Add the milk, bring to a boil, and cook for 3 minutes, or until the liquid has reduced by about half. Transfer the mixture to a 9 x 9-inch baking dish.

4. In a small bowl, stir together the cheese, almond flour, and oat bran and scatter over the squash. Bake for 15 minutes, or until the top is lightly browned and the liquid in the pan is bubbling.

Per serving: 127 calories • 7g protein • 8.5g fat (2g saturated) • 2g fiber • 8g carbohydrate • 316mg sodium • 48mg magnesium

If you have gluten issues: Choose a gluten-free brand of oat bran.

Gingered Butternut Squash and Carrot Puree

Hands-On Time: 20 minutes | **Total Time:** 40 minutes | **Makes:** 6 (½-cup) servings

If soup is your thing, add 2 cups low-sodium chicken or vegetable broth to the puree when reheating (you can use the liquid from step 1 of this recipe), and you've got a nice pot of butternut squash and carrot soup. Gut-soothing ginger is a key ingredient in this flavorful dish. Look for ginger that is plump in its skin, not at all withered, and store in the refrigerator if you'll be using it within a week or so. But for longer storage, peel the ginger, pop it in a resealable plastic bag, and freeze it—then when you need it, just grate the frozen ginger into your recipe.

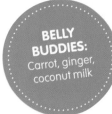

BELLY BUDDIES:
Carrot, ginger, coconut milk

3 cups peeled butternut squash in small chunks (about 1¼ pounds)

1 large carrot (8 ounces), thinly sliced

½ cup water

¼ cup thinly sliced peeled fresh ginger

1 teaspoon ground cinnamon

½ teaspoon ground cardamom

¼ teaspoon ground allspice

¾ teaspoon salt

½ cup light coconut milk

1. In a large saucepan, combine the squash, carrot, water, ginger, cinnamon, cardamom, allspice, and ¼ teaspoon of the salt. Bring to a boil, reduce to a simmer, cover, and cook for 20 minutes, or until the vegetables can be pierced with the tip of a knife.

2. Drain the mixture (reserve the liquid if you want to make a soup as described above) and transfer to a food processor. Add the coconut milk and the remaining ½ teaspoon salt and puree until smooth. Return to the saucepan and reheat over medium-low heat.

3. Serve hot or at room temperature.

Per serving: 77 calories • 1g protein • 1.5g fat (1g saturated) • 3.5g fiber • 16g carbohydrate • 325mg sodium • 39mg magnesium

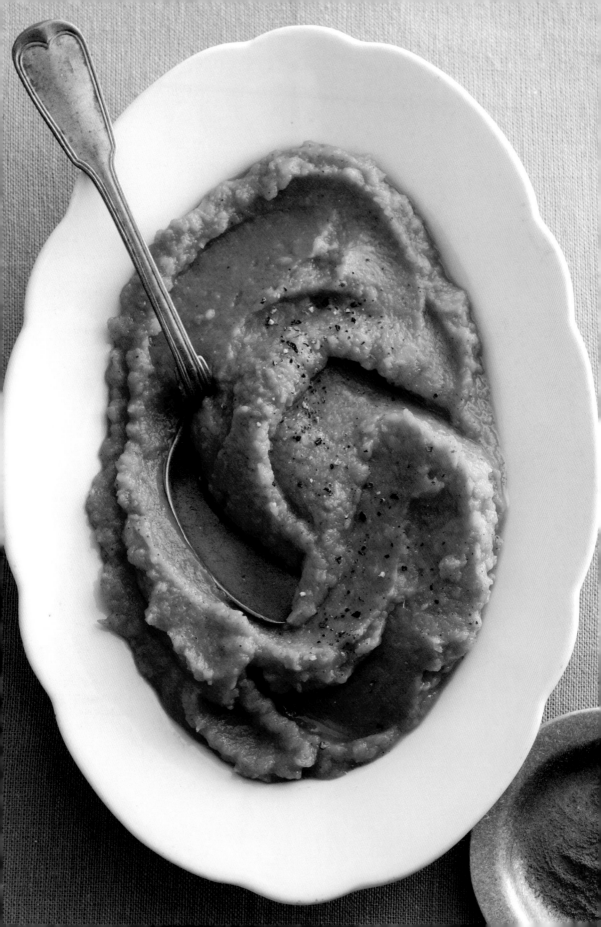

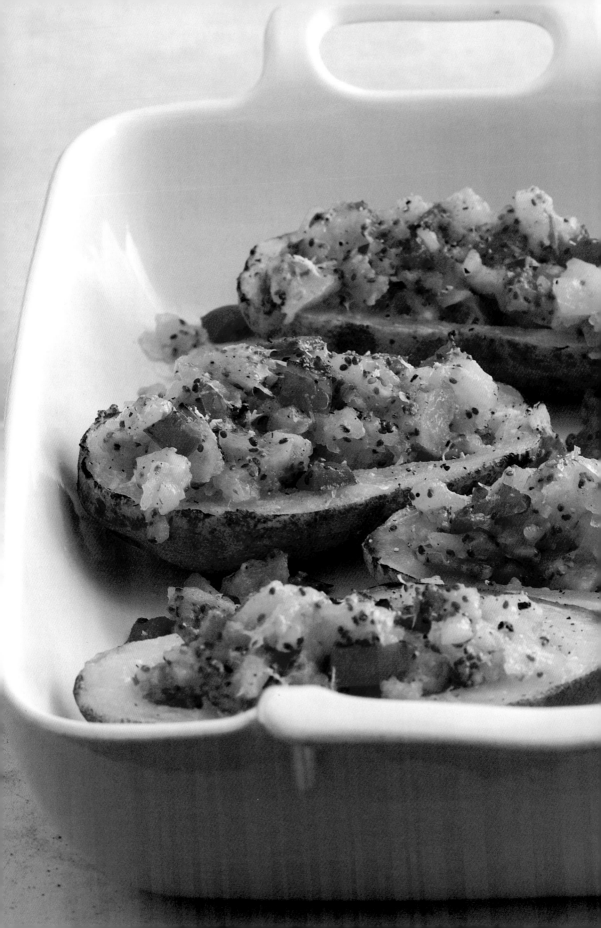

Twice-Baked Potatoes with Pepper Hash

Hands-On Time: 20 minutes | **Total Time:** 30 minutes | **Makes:** 4 servings

A delicious make-ahead side dish: Just prepare the stuffing, fill the potatoes, sprinkle with cheese, cover, and refrigerate. Reheat them for about 20 minutes in a 350°F oven before broiling the tops to brown the cheese.

2 russet (baking) potatoes (8 ounces each)

2 teaspoons Roasted Garlic Oil (page 211) or extra-virgin olive oil

2 teaspoons chia seeds

1 large red bell pepper, diced

¼ teaspoon salt

¼ teaspoon black pepper

¼ cup plus 2 tablespoons grated Parmesan cheese

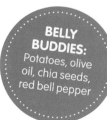

BELLY BUDDIES: Potatoes, olive oil, chia seeds, red bell pepper

1. Pierce the potatoes and microwave on high for 7 to 10 minutes (depending on the oven), or until firm-tender. Let sit for 2 minutes, then halve lengthwise and set aside until cool enough to handle.

2. Meanwhile, in a medium nonstick skillet, heat the oil over medium-high heat. Add the chia seeds and cook for 1 minute to toast. Add the bell pepper, salt, and black pepper and cook for 3 to 5 minutes, or until softened.

3. Preheat the broiler.

4. Scrape the potato flesh into a bowl, leaving a ¼-inch shell behind. Add the bell pepper mixture and ¼ cup cheese to the bowl and mash in.

5. Place the potato shells on a baking sheet. Spoon the filling back into the potato shells. Sprinkle with the 2 tablespoons cheese and broil for several minutes to brown the cheese.

Per serving: 163 calories • 6g protein • 5g fat (1.5g saturated) • 3g fiber • 24g carbohydrate • 268mg sodium • 40mg magnesium

If you have gluten issues: Choose a gluten-free brand of chia seeds.

Nutty Red Quinoa

Hands-On Time: 10 minutes | **Total Time:** 30 minutes | **Makes:** 4 (¾-cup) servings

Red quinoa is more robust than regular quinoa, and here it is nicely contrasted with sweet and tangy pineapple and crunchy pecans. Serve alongside Salmon with Preserved Lemon Topping (page 179) and steamed green beans. If you'd like, swap in orange segments for the pineapple.

BELLY BUDDIES:
Quinoa, olive oil, pineapple, pecans

- ⅔ cup red quinoa
- 3 teaspoons Roasted Garlic Oil (page 211) or store-bought garlic-infused oil
- ½ cup thinly sliced scallion greens or chives
- ½ teaspoon salt
- ¼ teaspoon black pepper
- ⅔ cup canned pineapple chunks in 100% pineapple juice, drained and halved
- ⅓ cup pecans, coarsely chopped

1. In a small bowl, combine the quinoa with cold water to cover by 2 inches. Let sit for 2 minutes. Swish around and drain the water off (leave the quinoa in the bowl). Add fresh water to cover by 2 inches and let sit for 5 minutes. Drain well in a fine-mesh sieve.

2. In a small saucepan, heat 1½ teaspoons of the oil over medium heat. Add the scallion greens, stirring to coat. Add the quinoa, salt, pepper, and 1⅔ cups water and bring to a boil. Reduce to a simmer, cover, and cook for 15 to 17 minutes, or until the quinoa is tender.

3. Transfer to a bowl and stir in the pineapple, pecans, and the remaining 1½ teaspoons oil. Serve warm, at room temperature, or chilled.

Per serving: 214 calories • 5g protein • 11g fat (1g saturated) • 3g fiber • 26g carbohydrate • 298mg sodium • 17mg magnesium

Sesame Pasta

Hands-On Time: 10 minutes | **Total Time:** 25 minutes | **Makes:** 4 (1-cup) servings

A good trick to soften the peanut butter for mixing in with the pasta (especially if you keep your peanut butter in the fridge) is to assemble the peanut butter and other dressing ingredients in a metal bowl that you can set over the cooking pasta. The heat will soften up the peanut butter. I like using radiatore pasta for this recipe because the ridges hold more of the sauce, but any type of gluten-free pasta will do. Grill some shrimp (about 6 ounces per person) and either serve them alongside the pasta or cut them up and toss them with the pasta and peanut sauce.

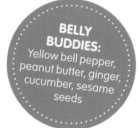

BELLY BUDDIES: Yellow bell pepper, peanut butter, ginger, cucumber, sesame seeds

- 4 ounces gluten-free pasta
- ½ teaspoon salt
- 1 yellow bell pepper, cut into ½-inch squares
- 2 tablespoons natural peanut butter
- 1 tablespoon reduced-sodium soy sauce
- 1 tablespoon rice vinegar
- 2 teaspoons grated fresh ginger
- 1 cucumber, peeled, seeded, and cut into ½-inch chunks
- 2 teaspoons sesame seeds, toasted

1. Cook the pasta according to package directions, using the ½ teaspoon salt. Add the bell pepper for the last 2 minutes. Scoop out about 1 cup of the pasta cooking water and then drain the pasta and peppers.

2. In a bowl, combine the peanut butter, soy sauce, vinegar, and ginger. Add the pasta and peppers (the hot pasta should melt the peanut butter). If the sauce seems at all tight, stir in a little of the reserved pasta cooking water to loosen it up.

3. Stir in the cucumber. Serve sprinkled with sesame seeds.

Per serving: 189 calories • 5g protein • 5.5g fat (0.5g saturated) • 3.5g fiber • 31g carbohydrate • 178mg sodium • 21mg magnesium

If you have gluten issues: Choose a gluten-free brand of soy sauce.

Toasted Brown Rice and Pepper Pilaf

Hands-On Time: 5 minutes | **Total Time:** 1 hour | **Makes:** 6 (½-cup) servings

Leftovers of this pilaf would make a wonderful lunch salad: To ½ cup of the pilaf, add chopped cooked lean pork, turkey breast, or shrimp (about 3 ounces); 1 diced mini cucumber (also called Persian cucumber); 1 cup chopped watercress; and lemon or lime juice to taste.

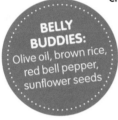

BELLY BUDDIES: Olive oil, brown rice, red bell pepper, sunflower seeds

- 2 teaspoons Roasted Garlic Oil (page 211) or extra-virgin olive oil
- 1 cup long-grain brown rice
- 1⅓ cups water
- ¾ cup carrot juice
- ½ teaspoon salt
- 1 large red bell pepper, finely diced
- 2 tablespoons hulled sunflower seeds or pumpkin seeds, chopped

1. In a saucepan, heat the oil over medium-high heat. Add the rice and stir to coat. Stir for 2 to 3 minutes to lightly toast.

2. Add the water, carrot juice, and salt. Bring to a boil, then reduce to a simmer, cover, and cook for 45 minutes, or until tender. Remove from the heat and let stand, covered, for 10 minutes.

3. Stir in the bell pepper and sunflower seeds and fluff with a fork.

Per serving: 165 calories • 4g protein • 4g fat (0.5g saturated) • 3g fiber • 29g carbohydrate • 220mg sodium • 61mg magnesium

Easy Belly-Friendly Salsa

Hands-On Time: 5 minutes | **Total Time:** 5 minutes | **Makes:** 4 (⅓-cup) servings

You probably already know to look out for sodium in your salsa, but trying to find an onion- or garlic-free variety is pretty tough. It's easy enough to make your own, though, especially if you use canned diced tomatoes rather than fresh.

1 can (14.5 ounces) no-salt-added diced tomatoes, juice drained (look for brands with no onions or garlic)

¼ cup chopped fresh cilantro

1 tablespoon lime juice

3 scallion greens, sliced thinly

Pinch of salt

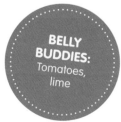

BELLY BUDDIES: Tomatoes, lime

In a medium bowl, add the tomatoes, cilantro, lime juice, scallions, and salt. Toss together and refrigerate.

Per serving: 24 calories • 1g protein • 0g fat (0g saturated) • 1g fiber • 5g carbohydrate • 249mg sodium • 2mg magnesium

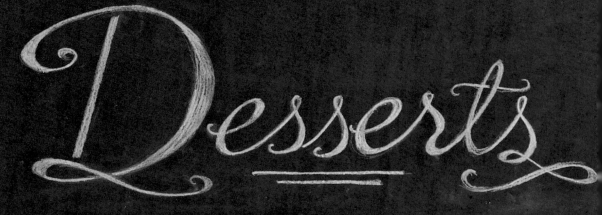

Desserts

SWEET ON BELLY BUDDIES!

MADE IN A
MUFFIN TIN!

SWEETENED
WITH
MAPLE SYRUP!

Almost-Pumpkin
Mini Pies~

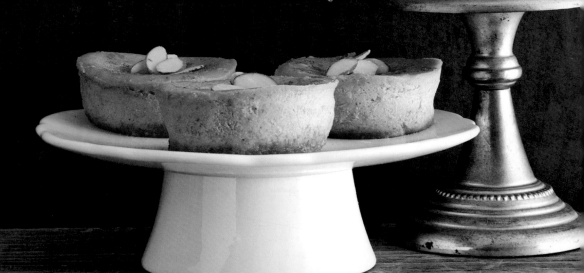

Almost-Pumpkin Mini Pies

Hands-On Time: 15 minutes | **Total Time:** 1 hour 10 minutes plus cooling | **Makes:** 6 mini pies

These days you can buy peeled and cut-up butternut squash in the supermarket—an incredible time-saver in the kitchen. The mini pies can be frozen and kept in an airtight container for up to 3 months. To serve, let thaw at room temperature. Don't try to reheat them to thaw.

1 pound peeled butternut squash chunks

3 ounces fat-free cream cheese

3 tablespoons pure maple syrup

2 large eggs

3 large egg whites (or ½ cup liquid egg whites)

¾ teaspoon ground cinnamon

½ teaspoon ground ginger

¼ teaspoon ground allspice

Pinch of grated nutmeg

3 tablespoons plus 2 teaspoons turbinado sugar

Salt

¼ cup almond flour

2 tablespoons ground flaxseed

2 tablespoons sliced almonds

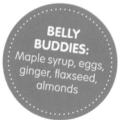

BELLY BUDDIES: Maple syrup, eggs, ginger, flaxseed, almonds

1. Preheat the oven to 350°F. Line 6 cups of a jumbo muffin tin with paper liners.

2. In a steamer, cook the squash for 10 to 15 minutes (depending on the size of the chunks), or until very tender. Spread the squash on several layers of paper towels and let sit for 10 minutes to cool slightly and release steam.

3. Transfer the squash to a food processor and add the cream cheese, maple syrup, whole eggs, egg whites, cinnamon, ginger, allspice, nutmeg, 3 tablespoons sugar, and ¼ teaspoon salt. Puree until very smooth.

4. In a bowl, stir together the almond flour, flaxseed, 2 teaspoons sugar, and a generous pinch of salt. Divide the mixture among the muffin cups (about 1 tablespoon per cup). With a small juice glass, press the mixture firmly into the bottom of the cups.

5. Divide the batter among the muffin cups. Bake for 40 minutes, or until puffed and lightly browned. Remove the "pies" from the pan and place on a rack to cool to room temperature (they will sink). Then refrigerate until well chilled.

6. To serve, carefully peel away the muffin liner. Sprinkle with a dash of cinnamon and slivered almonds.

Per mini pie: 190 calories • 9g protein • 6g fat (1g saturated) • 3g fiber • 28g carbohydrate • 277mg sodium • 54mg magnesium

Peanut Butter–Banana Freeze

Hands-On Time: 10 minutes | **Total Time:** 10 minutes plus freezing | **Makes:** 6 servings

Bananas and Greek yogurt, both high in magnesium, are a couple of the best buddies your belly could have. Your taste buds will thank you, too. You can also turn these into a chocolate-chip version: Don't melt the chocolate but fold finely chopped dark chocolate into the banana mixture.

BELLY BUDDIES:
Bananas, Greek yogurt, peanut butter

- 2 very ripe bananas (6 ounces each)
- ½ cup nonfat plain Greek yogurt
- ¼ cup natural peanut butter
- 1 tablespoon pure maple syrup
- 1 teaspoon vanilla extract
- 2 ounces dark chocolate, melted and cooled to room temperature

1. In a food processor, combine the bananas, yogurt, peanut butter, maple syrup, and vanilla and puree until smooth. Add the chocolate and pulse to combine.

2. Divide the mixture among 6 ice pop molds or six 4-ounce custard cups or ramekins. Freeze for at least 4 hours, or until firm. Unmold the pops or serve in the custard cups.

Per serving: 166 calories • 5g protein • 9g fat (3g saturated) • 2.5g fiber • 19g carbohydrate • 8mg sodium • 11mg magnesium

If you have gluten issues: Choose a gluten-free brand of Greek yogurt.

Blueberry "Custard"

Hands-On Time: 20 minutes | **Total Time:** 20 minutes plus cooling | **Makes:** 4 (1-cup) servings

Allspice and a little black pepper give this custard the slightest kick, while maple syrup heightens the sweetness of the berries. Check the label on the syrup you buy and be sure it's pure maple syrup, not "pancake syrup," which, among other ingredients, contains high-fructose corn syrup. Once opened, store the maple syrup in the fridge where it will keep indefinitely. Blueberries are a superfood loaded with disease-fighting antioxidants and anti-inflammation properties.

2 cups blueberries

3 tablespoons pure maple syrup

¼ teaspoon ground allspice

¼ teaspoon ground cinnamon

⅛ teaspoon black pepper

1 tablespoon water

1 large egg

1 large egg white

1 tablespoon coconut oil, melted

1 cup nonfat plain Greek yogurt

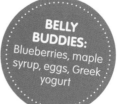

BELLY BUDDIES: Blueberries, maple syrup, eggs, Greek yogurt

1. In a small saucepan, combine the blueberries, maple syrup, allspice, cinnamon, pepper, and water. With a potato masher, gently mash the blueberries. Cook over medium heat, stirring frequently, for 7 minutes, or until the berries are very soft.

2. In a medium bowl, whisk together the whole egg, egg white, and coconut oil. Very gradually whisk the blueberry mixture into the egg mixture. Return the mixture to the saucepan and cook over medium-low heat, whisking constantly, for 4 minutes, or until the blueberry mixture has thickened. Transfer to a large bowl and let cool to room temperature.

3. Fold the yogurt into the cooled blueberries. Spoon into 4 serving bowls or goblets and refrigerate for 3 hours, or until well chilled.

Per serving: 164 calories • 8g protein • 5g fat (3.5g saturated) • 2g fiber • 23g carbohydrate • 55mg sodium • 10mg magnesium

If you have gluten issues: Choose a gluten-free brand of Greek yogurt.

Strawberry Soufflé-lets

Hands-On Time: 10 minutes | **Total Time:** 25 minutes | **Makes:** 6 servings

Any soufflés that won't be eaten right away can be saved and eaten later, although they will fall and condense—but the flavors will still be good. Take the "leftover" soufflés out of the muffin tin when they come out of the oven and let them cool on a rack.

BELLY BUDDIES:
Banana, strawberries, eggs

1 small ripe banana (6 ounces), cut up

4 ounces frozen strawberries, thawed

2 large eggs, separated

1 tablespoon turbinado sugar

1 tablespoon brown rice flour

1 egg white, at room temperature

Cream of tartar

3 teaspoons pure maple syrup

1. Position a rack in the lower third of the oven and preheat to 400°F. Line 6 cups of a jumbo muffin tin with paper liners.

2. In a mini food processor, process the banana and strawberries to a smooth puree. Add the egg yolks, sugar, and flour and process until smooth. Transfer to a large bowl.

3. In another bowl, with an electric mixer, beat the 3 egg whites with a generous pinch of cream of tartar until stiff peaks form. Scoop about one-third of the whites into the fruit mixture and whisk to lighten

the mixture. Gently fold in the remaining whites until no streaks of egg white show.

4. Divide the soufflé mixture among the muffin cups. Bake for 11 to 13 minutes, or until puffed and browned on top. To serve, transfer the whole muffin cup to a small ramekin. Poke a hole in the top of the soufflé and drizzle ½ teaspoon maple syrup down into the soufflé. Serve immediately.

Per serving: 82 calories • 3g protein • 2g fat (0.5g saturated) • 1g fiber • 14g carbohydrate • 34mg sodium • 13mg magnesium

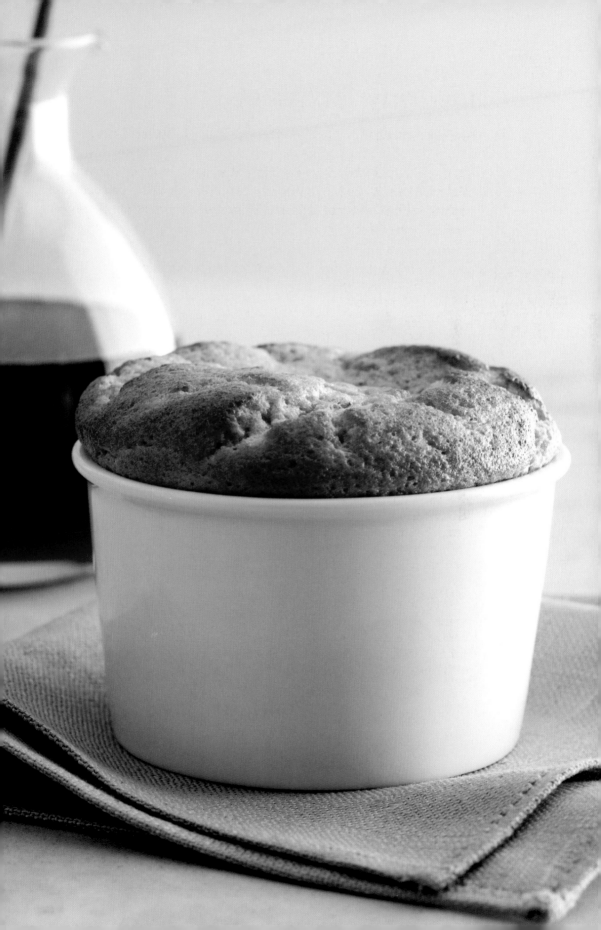

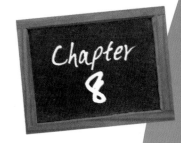

The 21-Day Tummy Workout

In my thirties, I worked as executive editor of *Fitness* magazine, where it was axiomatic that exercise was good for your weight, your waistline, your mood, your heart, your brain, your sex life, and on and on and on. So I wasn't surprised to learn recently that the right fitness routine is good for gut health, too.

Happily, the key to making a workout belly-friendly lies in just a few simple moves that don't take much time and don't require any equipment. Specially designed to blast ab fat, sculpt your stomach, and calm tummy troubles, the 21-Day Tummy workout is a perfect complement to your eating plan. While you can soothe and shrink your belly with the diet alone, you'll get results faster if you add on this easy and effective exercise routine.

A Moving Solution

By definition, the more physical activity you do, the more calories you burn. But that doesn't mean that the longer or harder you exercise, the more weight you lose. In fact, it turns out that strenuous exercise can backfire, sabotaging your weight-loss efforts. What's more, intense exercise may actually harm your digestive system. Moderate exercise, on the other hand, confers a plethora of benefits on your tummy.

The Problem with Exercising Too Much

Over the past few years, research has accumulated showing that the exercise–weight loss equation is far from linear. In a study of more than 400 postmenopausal women, researchers divided participants into three groups. One group exercised for about 10 minutes a day, one for about 20 minutes a day, and the third for almost 30 minutes a day. After 6 months, the women in the 20-minute-per-day group had lost an average of 50 percent more weight than those in the 10-minute-per-day group. But the women who exercised 30 minutes a day lost only 7 percent more than those who did 10 minutes a day—and they lost nearly 30 percent less than those who exercised for 20 minutes a day![1] See, after exercising a certain amount, you get hungry. So you eat more, usually consuming more calories than you burned.

Even worse, strenuous exercise appears to damage the intestinal lining, disturbing gut bacteria and allowing bacterial endotoxins to escape into the bloodstream. This restricts blood flow to the GI system, triggering inflammation.[2]

Inflammation, in turn, leads to many serious health issues, including weight gain and gastrointestinal issues. That explains why up to half of elite athletes, who train harder and longer than the rest of us, suffer from diarrhea, nausea, heartburn, and other GI symptoms.[3] Female athletes are more likely than male athletes to have stomach problems, and of all athletes, runners in particular fall prey to digestive discord most often, according to a study in *Sports Medicine*.[4]

The Benefits of Exercising Just Enough

To get results, then, you don't want to spend hours on the treadmill—which I'm sure you weren't planning to do anyway! Instead, most research points to about 20 minutes a day of moderate activity as optimal for a slim and calm belly. How do shorter bursts of regular movement help your tummy?

Moderate exercise slashes dangerous belly fat. A study conducted at Saint Louis University showed that exercise worked better than calorie restriction to reduce dangerous visceral fat.[5] In another study, Japanese women who performed short bouts of physical activity throughout the day had less visceral fat.[6]

> Strenuous exercise can backfire, sabotaging your weight-loss efforts. Moderate exercise confers a plethora of benefits.

Moderate exercise keeps the pounds off for life. The National Weight Control Registry, a database of people who have lost at least 30 pounds and kept it off for at least a year, reports that an astonishing 94 percent of participants increased their physical activity as a way of maintaining their weight loss success.[7]

Moderate exercise moves intestinal muscles. In Chapter 2, I described the powerful muscles in your digestive tract that are crucial to keeping things moving along down there. You may not feel it, but exercise helps the muscles in your gut just like the ones you see in your arms, legs, and butt. When you exercise, your heart starts pumping faster, increasing blood flow and oxygen circulation to cells throughout your body, including your intestinal muscles. This stimulates peristalsis, the wavelike motion that moves food through your digestive tract.

Moderate exercise improves digestive symptoms. In a 2011 Swedish study, 102 IBS patients were split into two groups. One was instructed to increase their physical activity to 20 to 30 minutes three to five times a week. The other group continued the same habits as before. After 3 months, the participants rated their IBS symptoms. The group that had increased their exercise time experienced fewer symptoms.[8]

Moderate exercise stops inflammation in its tracks. In a study of elderly Japanese women, for instance, just 12 weeks of resistance training significantly reduced levels of C-reactive protein, an inflammatory marker, in the bloodstream.[9] The same thing held true for young, healthy women in a study conducted by Louisiana State University who did a combination of endurance and resistance training.[10]

Moderate exercise reduces stress. When you exercise, your body produces endocannabinoids, your brain's natural feel-good substances (and yes, they are chemically similar to cannabis, or marijuana).[11] Exercise also reduces the levels of the stress hormones adrenaline and cortisol.

The Triple Threat of the 21-Day Tummy Workout

Any kind of movement can help fend off visceral fat, digestive issues, and other health problems. But research points to some specific types of exercise that are especially good for your belly. We've built the three-pronged 21-Day Tummy workout around these: interval walking, core strength training, and yoga.

To put together this slimming, calming, and tummy-toning exercise routine, I turned to Michele Stanten, an American Council on Exercise certified fitness trainer who is well versed in the research on what exercises are best for bellies. A walking expert and longtime yoga practitioner, she's the best person I know to combine these different types of exercise into a simple, practical routine that anyone can do.

Interval Walking

Walking is the number one exercise of choice for most North Americans—and for good reason. It's easy, it doesn't require much equipment, and you can do it pretty much anywhere. As part of my commute, I walk about an hour a day round-trip to and from the train, and it's amazing how much better I feel just from this simple exercise.

But there's a big difference between a leisurely stroll around the block and a brisk hike up a mountain. At higher intensities, you are burning more calories and training your heart and lungs to work at a higher capacity. Because most of us can't keep up the pace for too long—and working too hard for too long causes digestive distress—we need a compromise: interval walking.

> Research shows that interval training is tops at burning belly fat.

The principle is simple: By alternating intervals of high intensity activity and low intensity activity, you can go longer than you could at the high intensity but you'll burn more calories than you could at the low intensity. Plus, by adding variety to your workout, you're less likely to get bored—and more importantly, your body is less likely to adapt and your weight loss less likely to plateau.

After an interval training session, your body breaks down more stored fat.[12] This is called fat oxidation, and it's usually what your body does when it's ready to take fat out of storage to burn it. Even if your body doesn't actually burn this fat, just breaking it down causes it to take up less space so you look slimmer. Also, exercisers are generally less hungry after interval training sessions because levels of the hunger hormone ghrelin drop.[13]

Finally, research shows that interval training is tops at burning belly fat—both the subcutaneous kind that jiggles and wiggles and the visceral kind that can cause deadly disease. In a French study, men who did an interval workout just once a week (along with endurance training twice a week) for

8 weeks slashed their belly fat by 44 percent![14] In an earlier study, participants following a similar exercise regimen (endurance training twice a week and interval training once a week) dropped visceral fat by 48 percent and subcutaneous fat by 18 percent.[15]

Michele based the 21-Day Tummy interval workout on these two studies because, of all the research on interval training, they demonstrated the greatest percentage of abdominal fat loss. In both, the intervals are on the longer side (2 minutes of high intensity activity for every 3 minutes of low intensity activity) and the high intensity activity kept at 75 to 85 percent of peak oxygen uptake. That means the study participants weren't going 100 percent as fast or as hard as they could, even during the high intensity intervals. Similarly, while you'll be working harder during your high intensity intervals, you won't be walking flat out. This allows you to avoid the superstrenuous exercise that can cause digestive discord.

> Strength training is the only way to sculpt the toned tummy you want.

Core Strength Training

While aerobic exercise, such as walking, running, cycling, or swimming, has proven to be the most effective for weight loss, strength training is also key to a flat stomach.

First, muscles burn calories even when you're not actively using them. This is what people mean when they say building muscle boosts metabolism. Also, fat oxidation increases after strength training, as your body takes fat out of storage to burn. At the same time, your body uses oxygen to replenish your fat. That's known as excess postexercise oxygen consumption, or EPOC, and it also burns calories. While it turns out the net calorie burn from both of these effects is relatively small, it is real and I believe every little bit helps.

More importantly, strength training reduces inflammation. Remember the studies I shared with you earlier about how levels of inflammatory markers dropped after moderate exercise? They all used resistance training. By now, you know just how lowering inflammation can help shrink and soothe your belly.

Finally, strength training is the only way to sculpt the toned tummy or six-pack abs you want. In addition to working those surface abdominal muscles (the rectus abdominis), you want to reach the deeper muscles of the waist and back that help to stabilize your spine and improve your posture, which in turn helps your belly look flatter.

That means we're not going to have you do endless sit-ups or crunches. In fact, sit-ups only work the rectus abdominis, so they're not very effective at strengthening your whole core. Instead, Michele has focused on moves that work multiple muscle groups at once so you get a full core strengthening routine with just five simple exercises.

BREATHE FOR BETTER DIGESTION

It's not just in yoga that you need to pay attention to your breathing. During each workout, think about your breath supporting your movement and helping to settle your stomach. Calm any anxious flutters with one of these exercises:

1. **Gentle Breath:** Sit in a comfortable position. Inhale deeply and as slowly as possible through your nose, with your mouth closed. Imagine getting the air deep into your stomach. If you put a hand on your stomach, you should feel your stomach expand. Hold this breath for 2 seconds. Exhale through your nose, seeing if you can make the exhale take as long as the inhale took. Your stomach should contract on the exhale. If your stomach is moving, you're breathing deeply. If only your chest is moving, you're breathing too shallowly. Continue this cycle for 1 minute or longer, if desired.

2. **Snap Breath:** Inhale deeply and as slowly as possible through your nose, with your mouth closed. Pause. On the exhale, force your breath out quickly through your nose, hard enough so that it feels like it's snapping from your stomach. The "snap" should be noticeable. Put one hand on your stomach to track it; your stomach should expand on the inhale and contract on the exhale. Repeat this cycle for 30 seconds, gradually increasing the pace of both the inhale and exhale as you become more comfortable with this technique.

Yoga

All types of exercise help to reduce stress, but yoga is an especially powerful stress-buster. As we learned in Chapter 2, chronic stress throws our hormones out of whack, causing us to crave fattening and tummy-troubling foods, as well as slowing down digestion. In a study conducted by researchers at the Thomas Jefferson Medical College, yoga lowered levels of the stress hormone cortisol in healthy volunteers after just one 50-minute session.[16]

Yoga can also reduce chronic inflammation. In a study from the All India Institute of Medical Sciences, 86 patients with chronic inflammatory diseases, such as colitis, were given a "yoga treatment" that included classic yoga postures, breathing exercises, stress management, group discussions, lectures, and individualized advice. This yoga treatment reduced the markers of stress and inflammation in as few as 10 days.[17] Two other studies demonstrated that yoga worked better than conventional treatments in reducing the gastrointestinal symptoms of people with IBS.[18, 19] Michele based the yoga routine in the 21-Day Tummy workout on the poses used in these studies.

> In one study, yoga treatment reduced markers of stress and inflammation in as few as 10 days.

One of the hallmarks of yoga is the yogic breath, a full deep breathing I consider to be a form of exercise in and of itself. Deep breathing is good for us because it promotes a complete oxygen exchange in the lungs. When you take a deep breath and exhale it, carbon dioxide stored in your lungs is expelled and replaced with oxygen, energizing all the cells of your body. With shallow breathing, not all the carbon dioxide is removed. In addition to a fuller oxygen exchange, deeper breaths can also slow the heartbeat, and that calmness stabilizes or decreases blood pressure and may relieve the stress and anxiety that impair digestion.

The 21-Day Tummy Workout

As a busy working mom herself, Michele understands how tough it can be to fit in fitness. While we all have to spend at least a little time thinking about and preparing food (even if it just means placing a call for takeout), exercise seems optional and carving out 20 minutes to take a walk can sometimes seem impossible. That's why Michele has designed the 21-Day Tummy workout to be every bit as efficient as your meal plan. The interval walks can take as little as 15 minutes, the core strength workout about 10 minutes, and the yoga routine only 5. As tester Tonya Carkeet noticed, "On the days that I don't want to exercise, I realize I can have it done sooner than I can come up with a reasonable excuse not to do it!"

Since you don't need any equipment (just a good pair of walking shoes), you can do this routine anywhere. I sometimes shut the door to my office and do a few yoga poses to relax in between meetings.

Of course, there are some days when we recommend longer walks or workouts, but there's a lot of flexibility for you to fit them in whenever you can. If it's easier for you to do your walking, strength, and yoga routines back-to-back while you're in the zone, that's great. But if you only have 5 minutes here, 10 minutes there, break up the routine into whatever pieces make sense for you.

The workouts are designed to get a little more challenging each week, so that you keep surprising your body and avoid plateaus. If you find that the progressions are too hard for you, though, feel free to stay at the lower level until you're ready. By the same token, if you find yourself with extra energy—as several of our testers did—and want to do a little more, by all means do so!

Here's an overview of what to expect:

THE 21-DAY TUMMY **WORKOUT**

WEEK 1:

Walks
- 2 days/week, 15-minute Interval Walking Workout
- 2 days/week, walk for 25 minutes at a moderate intensity
- On the remaining days, fit in at least 30 minutes of walking (you can break this into smaller chunks throughout the day)

Moves
- At least 2 days/week: Slim and Strengthen Core Routine
- At least 2 days/week: Better Belly Yoga Routine

WEEK 2:

Walks
- 2 days/week, 20-minute Interval Walking Workout
- 2 days/week, walk for 35 minutes at a moderate intensity
- On the remaining days, fit in at least 30 minutes of walking (you can break this into smaller chunks throughout the day)

Moves
- At least 3 days/week: Slim and Strengthen Core Routine
- At least 3 days/week: Better Belly Yoga Routine

WEEK 3:

Walks
- 2 days/week, 25-minute Interval Walking Workout
- 2 days/week, walk for 45 minutes at a moderate intensity
- On the remaining days, fit in at least 30 minutes of walking (you can break this into smaller chunks throughout the day)

Moves
- At least 3 days/week: Slim and Strengthen Core Routine with Challenge Yourself option, if possible
- At least 3 days/week: Better Belly Yoga Routine

Walk Your Belly Off!

I want you to get in the habit of walking every day. Does that seem like a lot to you? Consider this: You're already walking every day—to the car, around the house, with the dog. So adding a few extra steps or a little more speed to the activities you're already doing is an easy way to burn a few extra calories and shed another inch or two of belly fat.

You'll see that Michele has built three different types of walks into the workout (see box at left). The first are the all-important interval workouts we talked about, which are designed to blast abdominal fat. You'll do those two days a week. Then, for balance, two days a week, you'll do some longer moderate-intensity steady-pace walks. On the remaining days, just count up the walking you're already doing—if it adds up to 30 minutes, you're done. If not, take another lap around the office to talk to your coworker in person.

While we recommend walking for this portion of the workout, you can also do both the intervals and steady-pace workouts while running, cycling, swimming, or any other cardiovascular activity. You can even do it in your living room. For the high intensity intervals, jog in place, lifting your knees up high, or do jumping jacks. For the low intensity intervals, march in place or step side to side.

Here are the details on how to do the interval walks:

PELVIC FLOOR EXERCISES

Your pelvic floor muscles form a sling that holds your intestines, bladder, and other organs in place. They also help hold or release urine and feces. Strengthening your pelvic floor muscles can prevent incontinence and constipation. (Researchers believe that pelvic floor dysfunction—when your pelvic floor muscles are unable to adequately evacuate feces from your rectum—is actually the cause of most cases of chronic constipation.[20]) It also improves sexual function, a nice bonus! To train your pelvic floor muscles, simply tighten them as if you are stopping urine in midstream. Then relax them, as if to allow urine to flow again. Repeat as many times as you like. You can do this exercise on its own, or incorporate it into your Slim and Strengthen Core Routine or your Better Belly Yoga Routine any time you are holding a position, such as the Side Plank or Abdominal Twist.

Interval Walking Workout

WEEK 1

TIME	DURATION	ACTIVITY	DESCRIPTION
0:00	3 minutes	Warm-up	Walk at an easy pace to increase blood flow to your working muscles and prepare your body for more intense activity. Gradually increase to a moderate intensity by the end of the 3 minutes.
3:00	2 minutes	High intensity	Go faster. You should be working at about 75 to 85 percent of your maximum effort. You should be breathing harder and your heart should be beating faster. You should still be able to talk in brief phrases. If you can't talk or can only manage yes/no responses, ease up a bit. If you can speak in full sentences, push harder.
5:00	3 minutes	Low intensity	Slow down to a pace at which you can speak in full sentences. You should be working at about 50 to 60 percent of your maximum effort.
8:00	2 minutes	High intensity	(see above)
10:00	3 minutes	Low intensity	(see above)
13:00	2 minutes	Cooldown	Gradually slow down to an easy pace to bring your breathing and heart rate back to normal.
15:00		Finished	

WEEK 2

TIME	DURATION	ACTIVITY	DESCRIPTION
0:00	3 minutes	Warm-up	Walk at an easy pace to increase blood flow to your working muscles and prepare your body for more intense activity. Gradually increase to a moderate intensity by the end of the 3 minutes.
3:00	2 minutes	High intensity	Go faster. You should be working at about 75 to 85 percent of your maximum effort. You should be breathing harder and your heart should be beating faster. You should still be able to talk in brief phrases. If you can't talk or can only manage yes/no responses, ease up a bit. If you can speak in full sentences, push harder.
5:00	3 minutes	Low intensity	Slow down to a pace at which you can speak in full sentences. You should be working at about 50 to 60 percent of your maximum effort.

WEEK 2 (continued)

TIME	DURATION	ACTIVITY	DESCRIPTION
8:00	2 minutes	High intensity	(see above)
10:00	3 minutes	Low intensity	(see above)
13:00	2 minutes	High intensity	(see above)
15:00	3 minutes	Low intensity	(see above)
18:00	2 minutes	Cooldown	Gradually slow down to an easy pace to bring your breathing and heart rate back to normal.
20:00		Finished	

WEEK 3

TIME	DURATION	ACTIVITY	DESCRIPTION
0:00	3 minutes	Warm-up	Walk at an easy pace to increase blood flow to your working muscles and prepare your body for more intense activity. Gradually increase to a moderate intensity by the end of the 3 minutes.
3:00	2 minutes	High intensity	Go faster. You should be working at about 75 to 85 percent of your maximum effort. You should be breathing harder and your heart should be beating faster. You should still be able to talk in brief phrases. If you can't talk or can only manage yes/no responses, ease up a bit. If you can speak in full sentences, push harder.
5:00	3 minutes	Low intensity	Slow down to a pace at which you can speak in full sentences. You should be working at about 50 to 60 percent of your maximum effort.
8:00	2 minutes	High intensity	(see above)
10:00	3 minutes	Low intensity	(see above)
13:00	2 minutes	High intensity	(see above)
15:00	3 minutes	Low intensity	(see above)
18:00	2 minutes	High intensity	(see above)
20:00	3 minutes	Low intensity	(see above)
23:00	2 minutes	Cooldown	Gradually slow down to an easy pace to bring your breathing and heart rate back to normal.
25:00		Finished	

Slim and Strengthen Core Routine

This routine focuses on building core strength and muscle tone. If an exercise is too difficult, try the "Make It Easier" option. If you can complete all reps with good form, try the "Challenge Yourself" version. As you progress, it's OK to do some reps with one level and finish with another. You'll do this routine 2 or 3 days a week, for about 10 minutes each time (see box on page 240).

Side Plank with Knee Pull

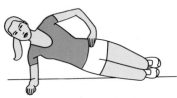

1. Lie on your right side with your legs bent and prop yourself up on your right forearm, elbow beneath your shoulder. Raise your hips off the floor.

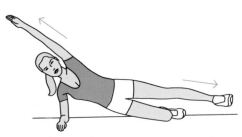

2. Inhale and extend your left leg and left arm, so that your left leg hovers a few inches above your right knee and your left arm is raised above your head.

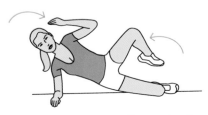

3. Bend your left arm and leg and pull your elbow and knee toward each other, contracting the left side of your torso as you exhale. Extend and repeat. Do 10–20 times, then repeat on the opposite side.

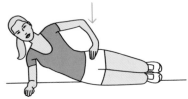

Make It Easier: Skip the knee pull in steps 2 and 3. Instead, simply hold the side plank position pictured in step 1, balancing on your right elbow and right lower leg with your thighs, hips, and torso off the floor. When you can hold each side for at least a minute, add a hip lift (pictured above): Lower and lift hips off the floor 10–20 times (pictured above), then repeat with the opposite side.

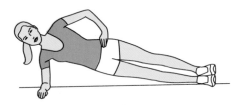

Challenge Yourself: After completing the recommended number of reps, extend your legs (with your feet stacked on top of each other) and hold a full side plank, working up to 1 minute on each side. When you can do that, try doing the knee pull while holding a full side plank.

All-Fours Crunches

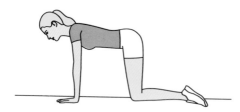

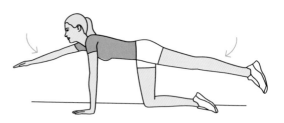

1. Get down on all fours with your hands beneath your shoulders and your knees beneath your hips.

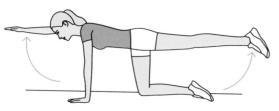

2. Inhale and raise your right arm out in front of you and your left leg behind you so your arm and leg are in line with your spine.

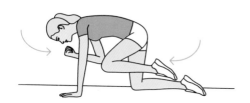

3. Exhale as you contract your abs, bend your right arm and left leg, and pull your elbow and knee toward each other. Extend your arm and leg and repeat the crunches. Do 10–20 times, then repeat with the opposite arm and leg.

Make It Easier: Skip the crunches in step 3 and simply hold the position pictured in step 2 with your right arm and left leg extended. When you can hold each side for at least a minute, add an arm and leg lift (pictured above): Lower your right arm and left leg to the floor, keeping them both straight. Then lift your right arm and left leg back to the position in step 2, in line with your spine. Do this 10–20 times, then repeat with the opposite arm and leg.

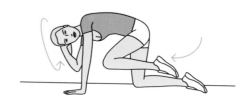

Challenge Yourself: In step 3, place your right hand behind your head. When you do your crunches, twist and pull your right elbow down toward your left knee.

Seated Rotation

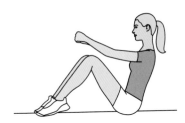

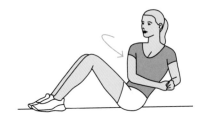

1. Sit on the floor with your legs bent, toes lightly touching the floor (but heels off the floor), and your arms in front of you with hands clasped.

Make It Easier: Perform the move with your feet flat on the floor and don't twist as far.

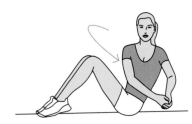

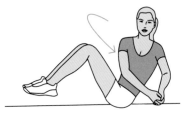

2. Inhale and then, as you exhale, contract your abs and slowly rotate your torso to the right, bringing your hands toward the floor. Your knees stay still. Return to the center on an inhale and then rotate to the left. Do 10–20 times to each side.

Challenge Yourself: Raise your feet a few inches off the floor and perform the move balancing on your sitting bones.

Bicycle

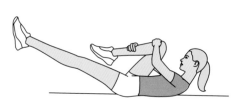

1. Lie on your back with your head and shoulders off the floor, your right knee pulled in toward your chest, and your left leg extended and about 15 inches off the floor.

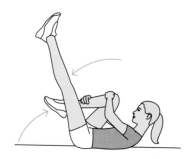

Make It Easier: Extend your leg toward the ceiling, at a 45-degree angle or greater, instead of straight ahead. Perform the move at this angle.

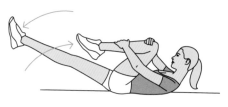

2. Inhale and switch legs, keeping your head and shoulders raised. Exhale and switch legs again, keeping your head and shoulders raised. Do 10–20 times with each leg.

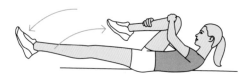

Challenge Yourself: Lower your extended leg so it's just a few inches off the floor. Perform the move at this angle.

Facedown Arm Lifts

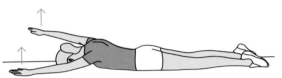

1. Lie facedown with your arms extended in a V shape. Squeeze your shoulder blades together and raise your arms a few inches off the floor as you inhale.

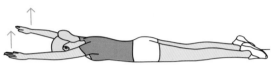

Make It Easier: Do the lifting and lowering part in step 1 and 3 only, skipping the pull back portion in step 2.

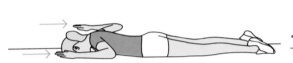

2. Exhale as you bend your elbows and pull your arms back so your hands are by your head, squeezing your shoulder blades tighter.

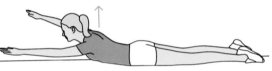

Challenge Yourself: Lift your head and chest off the floor as you do the move.

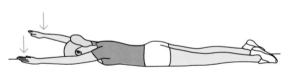

3. Extend your arms back into a V shape, keeping them a few inches off the floor, as you inhale. Lower your arms to the floor, keeping them in a V shape, as you exhale. Do 10–20 times.

Better Belly Yoga Routine

This routine features yoga poses that can lower stress, thus soothing digestive problems and preventing the development of belly fat. The whole sequence takes only about 5 minutes, 2 to 3 days a week (see box on page 240). But you can always do more if you find it helpful. If you find a pose that really helps relieve your tummy, you can also simply do that pose any time you notice GI symptoms. Listen to your body and move within a comfortable range of motion.

Forward Bend

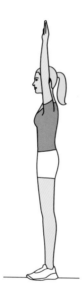

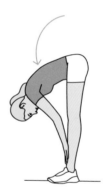

1. Stand with your feet together. Take a deep breath in and raise your arms overhead.

2. Exhale and bend forward, hinging from your hips, not your waist, and reaching your arms forward as you lower. Place your hands on your thighs, shins, or floor, whichever is most comfortable.

3. Inhale and lift your chest and head, lengthening your spine.

4. Exhale and round your back. Hold this position as you take 3 to 5 deep breaths. Relax and think about stretching your head toward the floor and bringing your chest closer to your legs with each breath. You can bend your knees slightly if needed.

5. Press into your hands and slowly roll up one vertebra at a time. Do this at least twice.

Cat Cow

1. Get down on all fours with your hands beneath your shoulders, your knees beneath your hips, and your head in line with your spine.

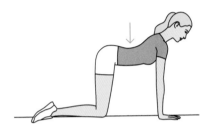

2. Inhale and lift your chest and tailbone toward the ceiling to arch your back.

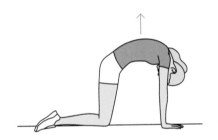

3. Exhale and round your back, tucking your tailbone and dropping your chin toward your chest. Do this for at least 5 deep breaths.

Rocking Hug

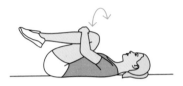

Lie faceup on the floor. Hug your knees into your chest and rock side to side, taking deep breaths as you rock. You can keep your head on the floor or lift it toward your knees. You can also try rocking forward and back, tucking your chin into your chest and lifting your head and shoulders off the floor as you roll forward. Or simply hold the position with your head and shoulders off the floor. Practice what feels best for you. If rocking, do at least 10 times; if holding, hold for at least 5 breaths.

Abdominal Twist

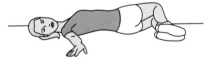

Lie faceup with your arms extended out to your sides and knees bent, feet flat on the floor. Slowly lower your knees to the left and look to the right, keeping your shoulders on the floor. Hold for at least 5 deep breaths, then switch sides.

***

That's it! Just five strength moves, four yoga poses, and three types of walks—seems almost too simple to work, right? But I promise it's not only efficient, it's effective. And you know what I like to say about exercise? Ninety percent is just showing up. A body at rest tends to stay at rest, whereas a body in motion tends to stay in motion. So once you get over the initial inertia of getting your walking shoes, and just start moving, I bet you won't want to stop!

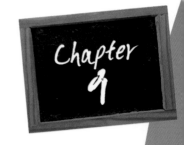

Terrific Tummy for Life

Congratulations! You've completed the 21-Day Tummy meal plan and, if you're anything like me and the rest of our testers, you feel fabulous. Your stomach is flatter, your gas pains and heartburn have disappeared, and you feel lighter, leaner, cleaner, and healthier. Maybe you've achieved the toned abs you've always wanted, or maybe you still have more weight to lose. Either way, you've taken a huge step toward a slim, calm, balanced belly.

For the last three weeks, you've eliminated any potentially problematic foods from your body. Now it's time to learn how to eat for life. You will systematically add foods back into your diet, but do it in a way that keeps you slim. This chapter will show you how to dodge the dreaded weight-loss plateau to finally get to your goal weight; add your favorite foods back to your diet without disturbing your tummy; and avoid regaining the pounds.

Get to Your Goal

Think back to the moment you picked up this book. What did you hope it would help you achieve? Were you mostly unhappy about the way your belly bulges? Or more concerned about the uncomfortable bloating you experience almost constantly? Was there a number on the scale you wanted to see? If you've accomplished all you wanted by this point, it's time to identify the foods that were specifically problematic for you, and which Belly Bullies you're able to eat.

To make sure you can eat the widest variety of foods and get all the nutrition you need, take the Belly Bully Tests to identify the foods that are a problem for you.

If you still have weight to lose, continue to enjoy the calorie-controlled, nutrient-balanced meals from any phase of the 21-Day Tummy eating plan. So you'll keep dropping the pounds while you challenge the Belly Bullies. When you know your test results you may be able to reintroduce healthy and satisfying foods like beans, blackberries, and barley that can help you stick to the diet over the long term.

Once you've finished the tests, repeat Phases 2 and 3 of the 21-Day Tummy meal plan. For variety, occasionally add in the Belly Bullies you've just discovered are safe for you. Continue doing that until you've reached your goal weight. I don't recommend going back to Phase 1 if you are continuing to lose weight. The lower calorie level in that phase can cause your body to believe it's starving. If you repeat this phase too often, your body holds on tighter to its fat stores.

If you are still experiencing digestive symptoms, cycle through Phases 2 and 3 until you are symptom-free. You should only need to repeat these two phases once in order to completely calm your tummy. But if your symptoms continue to bother you, start a food diary, noting exactly what you eat and when your symptoms appear. You may find that you've inadvertently gone off-plan and introduced a Belly Bully. If your food diary doesn't uncover an obvious tummy trigger, see your doctor; your symptoms may signal a more serious problem.

After you have been symptom-free for at least 3 days, take the Belly Buddy Tests to get a more precise sense of what's causing your problems and which Belly Bullies you can stand up to.

Identify Your Personal Belly Bullies

Many of the Belly Bullies we've identified are, in fact, very healthy. To make sure that you can eat the widest variety of foods and get all the nutrition you need, Kate has designed the Belly Bully Tests to pinpoint the foods that are a problem for you.

Note that carb-dense foods and pro-inflammatory fats affect everyone the same way, so you don't need to test them. Just keep your consumption to a minimum. The Belly Bully Tests we're presenting here will determine your sensitivity to specific FODMAPs. You may find your tolerance to different FODMAPs changes over time, due to changes in your gut bacteria, your stress level, your overall health, and other factors. So even if you fail a challenge now, it doesn't mean that food is off-limits forever. Repeat the test again in a few months.

Guidelines for the Belly Bully Tests

Here's how to identify your personal Belly Bullies:

- Take the tests one at a time. Remember to return to 21-Day Tummy clean eating after you've "passed" each.

- As you take each test, continue to follow the 21-Day Tummy meal plan (pick and choose your favorite meals from any phase). This will ensure you have limited intake of other potential offenders so it's clear what foods really bother you.

- Challenge the foods in the order provided.

- Consume the amount suggested in each Belly Bully test once per day for 2 to 3 days in a row (unless otherwise noted).

- Stop eating a food if you develop symptoms. Don't start your next test until you are symptom free for 2 to 3 days.

- Rechallenge a Belly Bully at a later date if you develop symptoms now.

- Track your tests with a food log such as this:

DAY/TEST	FOOD	QUANTITY	SYMPTOMS	

Test Doses for the Belly Bully Test

Here are the Belly Bullies you will be challenging over the next several weeks. Simply add the food described to your daily menu as you see fit. Remember, not all of these foods will be a Belly Bully for you; this is very individual.

TEST #1: Lactose

Drink 1 cup milk or eat 1 cup regular (not Greek) yogurt.

If your symptoms flare up after this challenge, avoid lactose-rich dairy products such as milk, yogurt, ice cream, custard, ricotta, and cottage cheese. Switch to lactose-free dairy versions of these foods. Most people digest hard cheeses well since they have less lactose. In fact, cheddar, Swiss and Parmesan cheeses are virtually lactose free. Greek yogurt is lower in lactose than regular yogurt, but if you're especially sensitive to lactose and you find that even the Greek yogurt gives you tummy trouble, substitute a lactose-free yogurt such as the Green Valley Organics brand.

You could also try lactase enzyme supplements. These enzymes can be purchased at your local drug store and will help your body break lactose down into its digestible sugars, glucose and galactose. When avoiding lactose-rich foods isn't an option, these lactase enzymes can come in handy!

TEST #2: Fructose

Eat ½ a mango or 1–2 teaspoons honey.

If you experience GI symptoms after this challenge, you will want to limit foods or beverages that contain more fructose than glucose. Remember, glucose helps your body digest fructose, and when there's too much fructose and not enough glucose, your digestive system may have problems. Examples of foods with a high fructose-to-glucose ratio include: apples, pears, mangoes, asparagus, sugar snap peas, honey, agave nectar, and any food containing high-fructose corn syrup.

TEST #3: Sorbitol (a type of polyol)

Eat 2 dried apricots or 1 nectarine.

If you fail the sorbitol challenge, avoid sugar-free gum and mints made with sorbitol, apples, pears, and stone fruits such as peaches, plums, and apricots.

TEST #4: Mannitol (a type of polyol)

Eat ½ cup mushrooms or ⅓ cup cauliflower.

If you fail the mannitol challenge, avoid mushrooms and cauliflower as well as mints and sugar-free gum made with mannitol.

TEST #5: Wheat (a source of fructans)

Eat 2 slices bread or 1 cup cooked pasta (consumed two to three times over the course of 1 week).

If wheat proves to be your downfall, try gluten-free breads, gluten-free pasta, and gluten-free cereals, since they won't contain wheat. Avoid beer and note that all types of breads and pastas, whether whole grain or white, have fructans.

TEST #6: Garlic (a source of fructans)

Eat 1 garlic clove (consumed two to three times over the course of 1 week).

If you find garlic doesn't suit you, replace it with the Roasted Garlic Oil recipe (page 211). Commercial soups and dressings often have garlic, so limit or avoid those as well.

TEST #7: Onion (a source of fructans)

Eat 1 tablespoon chopped onion (consumed two to three times over the course of 1 week).

If onions are your problem, try to replace them with the green part of scallions or perhaps some chives in your favorite onion-based recipes. Avoid commercially made salad dressings and soups, which are rich in onion ingredients.

TEST #8: GOS

Eat ½ cup kidney beans, soybeans (edamame), or black beans.

If beans bring on the gas, then simply minimize your bean intake. Canned lentils and chickpeas have lower amounts of GOS compared to other beans, so perhaps try small amounts such as ¼ cup on top of your salad, or use beans more as an accent to your meal than as a major part of it. Or try Beano, a digestive enzyme supplement that may help your body digest GOS more efficiently.

Through this process, many of our testers were able to identify exactly what was causing their GI problems. Milk was the most common culprit. Adrienne noticed symptoms after eating just one sugar-free breath mint. Polyols are one of her tummy triggers. Dorothy found that onions and bread, both sources of fructans, are the biggest culprits for her. "The heartburn and bloating comes back big time when I eat them." she noted ruefully. I had a terrible reaction after one squirt of agave nectar in my tea. I suspected agave nectar disagreed with me and, sure enough, I malabsorb fructose. I now avoid apples, mangoes, and asparagus, and have forsaken even honey in my daily tea!

Some testers were just as gratified to see which of their favorite foods they could add back in. Tonya rejoiced that "onions and garlic sit well with me." And I'm relieved that lactose isn't a major trigger for me. Welcome back, skim milk and cheese!

Stay Slim and Calm for Life

Once you've reached your weight-loss and health goals and figured out your personal tummy triggers, you're ready to create your personalized plan for a trim, trouble-free tummy for life. To maintain your healthy weight while keeping digestive discord at bay, you can continue to follow Phase 3 of the

21-Day Tummy meal plan, in which Kate has carefully balanced your plate with the optimal proportions of lean protein, healthy fats, and fiber-rich carbs. But let's give you some modifications so you don't get bored. Variety also guarantees that you get a good assortment of antioxidants, phytochemicals, and other nutrients. Here's how:

- Continue to eat three meals and one snack per day, spacing them about 2 to 3 hours apart.

- Mix and match meals and recipes from any phase, including the additional recipes in Chapter 7.

- Begin eating the FODMAPs you are not sensitive to. You can add them to the 21-Day Tummy recipes—if you find you can tolerate fructose, toss some sugar snap peas in with the **Herb-Roasted Shrimp (page 197)**; blend a little mango into your **Belly Smoother Smoothie (page 156)**; or serve some asparagus on the side with your **Grilled Turkey Cutlets with Grape Salsa (page 172)**. Pop some pistachios if fructans and GOS aren't a big problem for you. And if you're okay with the polyols, feel free to munch on fresh peaches and plums.

- Make sure to eat at least one magnesium-rich food a day such as chia seeds, flaxseeds, pumpkin seeds, brown rice, oats, peanuts and peanut butter, potatoes, spinach, and Swiss chard.

Make your own belly-friendly meals by designing a balanced plate that contains:

- **Colorful vegetables:** Fill half your plate with vegetables such as green beans, bean sprouts, carrot, cucumber, eggplant, endive, lettuce, parsnip, arugula, Swiss chard, spinach, turnip, tomato, or zucchini. It's hard to overdo it with vegetables, so pile them on! You'll want to stick mostly with Belly Buddies, but feel free to add in any FODMAP-containing vegetables, such as asparagus or artichoke, as long as they don't trigger symptoms for you.

- **Fiber-rich carbs:** Fill one-quarter of your plate with fiber-rich carbs such as oats, oat bran, brown rice, polenta, corn tortillas, quinoa, or a baked potato (with skin) to help keep your digestive system moving and to maintain your energy. Keep portions to the size of your fist. Remember that you want to continue to minimize carb-dense foods. A small roll or a handful of pretzels every once in awhile won't derail your progress, but no heaping plates of pasta, please!

- **Lean protein:** Fill one-quarter of your plate with lean proteins such as eggs, tofu, fish and other seafood, and lean cuts of chicken, turkey, or pork. These will keep your belly comfortably full. Keep portions to about the size of the palm of your hand.

- **Healthy fats:** Accent your meal with healthy fats such as walnuts, almonds, peanuts or peanut butter, chia seeds, flaxseeds, pumpkin seeds, olives, avocado, or olive oil to cool inflammation. Keep portions small, such as 2 tablespoons walnuts, almonds, or peanut butter; 2 teaspoons chia seeds; 1 tablespoon olive oil; 5 to 10 olives; or ⅛ avocado.

- Enjoy 2 to 3 servings of fruit per day, such as 1 cup berries, 1 banana, or 1 orange. You can have them as a snack or with one of your meals.

Finally, if you haven't been working out regularly, this is the perfect time to start. Remember, the National Weight Control Registry found that 94 percent of people use exercise to keep the pounds off. The 21-Day Tummy workout is an easy and effective way to get moving, but any kind of physical activity will help.

If your digestive symptoms start to flare up again or the pounds start to creep up, don't panic! Simply start the 21-Day Tummy plan over again from Phase 1 to calm and flatten your belly. (So that your body doesn't go into starvation mode, do this no more than 4 times per year.) I've done this a couple of times in the past year when I noticed some afternoon bloating, and I find it's an easy and quick way to feel lean and healthy. If you didn't exercise the first time around, add the 21-Day Tummy workout to speed your results.

> If your digestive symptoms start to flare up or the pounds start to creep up, don't panic!

Your Recipe for Happiness

After following the 21-Day Tummy diet, it's very possible that you'll feel not only lighter and healthier but also happier. Researchers at University College London studied more than 3,500 middle-aged office workers over 5 years and found that people who ate a diet high in fried food, processed food, fatty dairy products, and refined cereals had a 58 percent higher risk of depression than those who ate very few processed foods. On the flip side, study participants who ate the most whole foods—fruits, veggies, fish—had a 26 percent lower risk of future depression than those who ate the least whole foods.[1]

It makes perfect sense. Whole foods are bursting with in-gredients—omega-3 fatty acids, lean protein, smart carbs, and antioxidants—that have been shown to help ward off de-pression and anxiety, relieve stress, and boost mood. Those foods also help cool inflammation and right the balance of bacteria in our gut so that our tummies slim down and calm down. That's enough to make anyone happy.

***

The most important part of this diet—and an important part of life, in my opinion—is to feel good in your own skin. Less visceral fat, lower overall weight, and a trouble-free GI tract: These are ingredients to a longer, healthier, happier life.

Conclusion

Embedded in the walls of your digestive tract is a system of neurons so complex it's been called a second brain. In addition to controlling digestion, this branch of your nervous system may sense danger in your environment and even influence your mood. That's why people talk about following your "gut instincts" or "going with your gut."

Well, my gut is telling me that America needs this diet because it does something no other diet does: It tackles the biggest problems people have with their belly—including the tummy pooch everyone complains about and the constant heartburn, chronic constipation, and frequent gas and bloating no one will admit to.

21-Day Tummy is based on the latest science *and* the real-world feedback of yours truly and the rest of our test team. It works fast, it features delicious whole foods, and it can be followed anywhere. It will help you lose weight, improve your digestion, and reduce your risks of heart disease, cancer, type 2 diabetes, and many other inflammatory conditions. And it will make you happier.

I had a lot of fun on this journey because I was lucky enough to share the experience with our testers. I was inspired by them all, and I know you will be, too. Here's some of their best advice:

Rob McMahon: Commit to it 100 percent. It's easier than you think to reduce portions when you're eating the right kind of food. If you stick with it, you'll see results fast—I lost 9 pounds in just the first 5 days!

Gregg Roth: Be prepared to put in a little time to shop and prepare meals. The results are worth it.

Sabrina Ng: Try new foods and enjoy cooking! This plan will definitely make you feel better day to day.

Tonya Carkeet: Just get back on the plan and move forward if you mess up. Don't beat yourself up. Keep the focus on your ultimate goal. It took me a long time to get unhealthy; it will take a long time to get back.

Lauren Weiss: Learn the substitutions and plan ahead for eating out by checking the menu (online), eating wisely the whole day, and resisting temptations once you're at the restaurant.

Jonathan Bigham: Get support. I loved that our group shared their daily experiences and updates, so I knew I wasn't the only one having the same issues.

Adrienne Farr: Pay attention to how you feel and don't worry about the number on the scale. Once when I was almost done with the 21 days, I had a hard day. On top of that, a friend brought over pizza as a peace offering—now that's temptation. I had to freeze it so I wouldn't eat it. I looked in the mirror and I liked the changes I saw, so I decided to have tea instead. Ain't easy, but the discipline was worth it.

Me: Embrace the planning and food prep that's involved in the first weeks of the plan. The results you'll experinece are worth the investment of time and energy. I quickly lost the ten pounds that had crept onto my frame. And I now go through most days without even a hint of the pain and discomfort that had plagued me daily. Here's to your happy and healthy tummy!

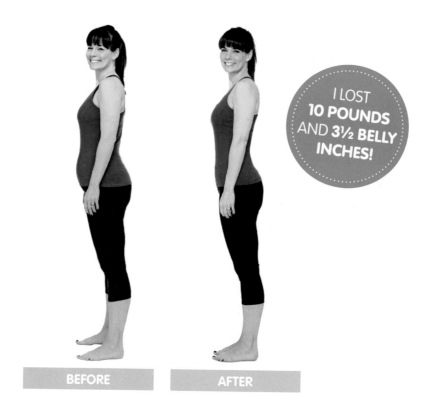

I LOST **10 POUNDS** AND **3½ BELLY INCHES!**

BEFORE

AFTER

Recipe Index

Weekly Shopping Lists

In order to make it easier for you to follow the 21-Day Tummy plan, we have compiled shopping lists for each week. These include the ingredients you would need if you are following the diet exactly as written. Keep in mind, however, that you may need to customize your shopping list depending on which recipes you use, which flavors you choose for your Belly Soother Smoothies, whether there are other people in your household you are cooking for, and if you make any food substitutions. Also, to save money, you may want to choose just one or two types of nuts, one or two types of salad greens, one type of olive oil (regular or extra virgin), one type of quinoa (red or regular), and so on. You'll see a few brands noted here, but also see page 152 for recommended brands of certain items.

Week 1 Shopping List

DAIRY

Greek yogurt, nonfat plain, one 32-ounce container plus three 6-ounce containers

Milk, nonfat lactose free (such as Dairy Ease or Lactaid), 1 quart

Mini cheeses, 1 mozzarella and 2 any kind (avoid cheese with added onion or garlic such as Laughing Cow Light)

Parmesan cheese, large container (either shredded or grated, or buy fresh and shred or grate your own)

MEAT/FISH/POULTRY

Beef, ground 93% lean, ¾ pound

Chicken breast, boneless skinless, 2 pounds

Pork, boneless center cut chop, 4 ounces

Salmon, 4 pieces (5 ounces each)

Shrimp, 6 large

Tuna, canned, packed in water, 5 ounces

White fish (halibut, cod, tilapia), 6 ounces

PRODUCE (Determine what smoothie flavors you intend to drink and add those fruits to your grocery list for the week)

Bananas, 2 small

Basil, 1 bunch

Bell pepper, 2 red

Blueberries, 1 pint

Bok choy, 1 bunch

Cantaloupe, 1 small

Carrots, 1 bag of baby and 1 small bag of regular size

Celery, 1 small bunch

Chives, 1 small bunch

Cilantro, 1 bunch

Dill, fresh, 1 bunch

Eggplants, 4 (8 ounces each)

Garlic, 12 cloves, about 3 heads

Ginger, fresh, 1 small piece

Grapes, red, 1 medium bunch

Green beans, ¾ pound

Green cabbage, 1 pound

Jalapeño chile pepper, 1

Kiwis, 4

Lemons, 2

Limes, 2

Orange, 1

Papaya, 1 small

Parsnips, 2

Red-skinned potatoes, 1¼ pounds

Romaine lettuce, 1 bunch

Russet (baking) potatoes, 2 pounds

Salad greens of choice, at least 6 cups (kale and/or spinach and/or arugula) (if you can find it, baby kale is more tender so it's a nice choice for salads)

Scallions, 1 bunch

Spinach, 1 large bunch

Strawberries, 1 pound

Sweet potato, 4 medium

Swiss chard, 1 bunch

Tomatoes, grape, 1 small box

Tomatoes, plum, 1½ pounds

Zucchini, 1 medium

NUTS/SEEDS

Almond butter, all natural, if desired for smoothies

Almonds, 1 bag whole plus 1 bag sliced

Chia seeds

Flaxseed, ground

Peanut butter, all natural (such as Smucker's, Teddie, or 365 Whole Foods)

Pecans

Pumpkin seeds

Sesame seeds

Walnuts

SPICES/PANTRY ITEMS

Balsamic vinegar

Basil

Black pepper, ground

Cinnamon

Coconut milk, light, 1 can

Cumin

Curry powder (look for brands with no onion or garlic, such as Spice Appeal)

Dijon mustard

Garlic-infused oil

Maple syrup, 100% pure

Olive oil, regular and extra-virgin

Paprika

Peanut oil

Quinoa, red, 1 package

Red wine vinegar

Rice vinegar

Sea salt

Sesame oil

Soy sauce, reduced sodium

Tomatoes, crushed, no-salt-added, 1 can (14.5 ounces; look for brands with no onions or garlic, such as Hunt's plain canned tomatoes or Muir Glen fire-roasted canned tomatoes)

Vanilla extract or paste

If choosing **CURRIED CHICKEN SOUP** recipe, add the following to your grocery list:

Bay leaf

Carrots, 4

Chicken breasts, 2 bone-in, skinless (8 ounces each)

Chicken broth, reduced sodium, 1 quart (or make your own)

Green beans, 1¼ pounds

Parsley

Thyme

Light spreadable cheese, 2 wedges (¾ ounce each)

Unsalted peanuts, small container

If choosing **CALDO VERDE** recipe, add the following to your grocery list:

Chicken broth, reduced sodium, 1 quart plus 1 14.5-ounce can

Dry white wine, small bottle

Hot paprika

Kale leaves, 8-ounce bunch

Lemon, 1

Red potatoes, 2 medium, (about ¾ pound)

Smoked ham, all-natural uncured, 4 ounces

White turnips, 2 medium (about ¾ pound)

Week 2 Shopping List

** = may have these item leftover from previous shopping week

DAIRY

Cheddar cheese, reduced fat, shredded, 1 bag

Cottage cheese, low-fat lactose-free, 1 small container

Cream cheese, ⅓ less fat, 1 small block (need 1 ounce)

Egg whites, 1 cup liquid or 6 large egg whites

Eggs, 6

Greek yogurt, nonfat plain, 2 containers (32 ounces each)

Greek yogurt, nonfat vanilla, 1 container (6 ounces)

Light spreadable cheese, 2 wedges (¾ ounce each)

Milk, nonfat lactose free (such as Dairy Ease or Lactaid), ½ gallon

Mini cheeses: 1 mozzarella and 2 any kind (avoid cheese with added onion or garlic such as Laughing Cow Light)

Parmesan cheese, grated or shredded **

MEAT/FISH/POULTRY

Chicken breast, bone-in, skin-on, 4 (10 ounces each)

Chicken breast, boneless, skinless, 1 pound

Pork, boneless center cut chop, 5 ounces

Pork tenderloin, 1 pound

Salmon fillet, 5 ounces

Shrimp, 6 large

Tuna steaks, 4 (5 ounces each)

PRODUCE (Determine what smoothie flavors you intend to drink
and add those fruits to your grocery list for the week)

Arugula, 2 bunches

Bananas, 1 bunch

Basil**

Bean sprouts, 1 bag

Belgian endive, 1

Bell pepper, 5 red and
  1 yellow

Blueberries, 1 pint

Boston lettuce, 1 head

Carrots, 1 bag of baby
  and 1 small bag of
  regular size**

Cantaloupe, 1 small**

Celery, 1 small bunch

Chives, 1 bunch**

Cucumber, 1 large

Garlic, 12 cloves,
  about 3 heads

Grapes, red, 1 medium
  bunch

Kiwi, 1

Lemons, 2

Lime, 1

Oranges, 3

Papaya, 1 medium

Parsley, 1 bunch

Pineapple chunks,
  in own juice (small
  can)

Pineapple, fresh, 1

Potato, 1 medium
  (Yukon Gold or
  red-skinned)

Raspberries, 1 pint

Roasted red pepper,
  1 jar (or get one at a
  salad bar)

Romaine lettuce,
  2 large heads

Scallions, 1 bunch

Spinach (frozen)
  2 boxes (10 ounces
  each)

Strawberries, 1 pint

Sunflower sprouts
  or pea shoots,
  1 container

Swiss chard, 1 large
  bunch

Tangerines, 2 large

Tomatoes, crushed,
  no-salt-added, 1 can
  (look for brands with
  no onions or garlic)

Tomatoes, grape,
  1 small container**

NUTS/SEEDS

Almond butter

Almonds, whole and
  sliced **

Chia seeds**

Peanut butter, all
  natural (such as
  Smucker's, Teddie,
  or 365 Whole
  Foods)**

Peanuts, unsalted

Pecans

Sesame seeds**

Walnuts**

SPICES/PANTRY ITEMS

Balsamic vinegar**

Black pepper, ground**

Cayenne pepper

Chicken broth, reduced sodium, 2 cans (14.5 ounces each)

Chili powder (look for brands with no onion or garlic, such as Spice Appeal)

Cinnamon**

Coconut milk, light, 1 can

Coconut oil

Curry powder (look for brands with no onion or garlic, such as Spice Appeal)**

Dijon mustard**

Dill

Garlic-infused oil**

Green olives, 1 jar

Kosher salt

Mandarin oranges, 1 small can, in 100% fruit juice

Maple syrup, 100% pure **

Mayonnaise, olive oil based

Oat bran (such as Bob's Red Mill or Quaker)

Olive oil, regular, extra-virgin,** and spray

Paprika**

Peanut oil**

Quinoa, red, 1 package**

Red wine vinegar**

Rice vinegar**

Sea salt**

Sesame oil**

Soy sauce, reduced sodium**

Turmeric

Water chestnuts, 2 cans (8 ounces each), sliced

Week 3 Shopping List

** = may have these item leftover from previous shopping week

DAIRY

Cheddar cheese, reduced fat, shredded, 1 bag**

Cottage cheese, low fat lactose free, 1 small container**

Greek yogurt, nonfat plain, 1 32-ounce and 1 6-ounce container

Greek yogurt, nonfat vanilla, 1 container (6 ounces)

Egg whites, 1 cup liquid or 6 large egg whites

Eggs, 6

Feta cheese, 1 small container or block

Milk, nonfat lactose free (such as Dairy Ease or Lactaid)

Mini cheeses, 1 mozzarella and 2 any kind (avoid cheese with added onion or garlic such as Laughing Cow Light), 8 ounces, 1 package **

MEAT/FISH/POULTRY

Chicken breast, boneless, skinless, 1 pound

Chicken, ground, 8 ounces

Fish (cod, haddock or tilapia), 4 ounces

Flank steak, 1¼ pounds

Pork, boneless center cut chop, 4 ounces

Tuna, canned, packed in water, 5 ounces

Turkey, deli, 4 slices

Turkey, ground, 1¼ pounds

PRODUCE (Determine what smoothie flavors you intend to drink and add those fruits to your grocery list for the week)

Bananas, 1 bunch

Basil**

Bell pepper, 3 red and 1 yellow

Blueberries, 1 pint

Bok choy, 1 bunch

Cantaloupe, 1 small

Carrot juice, 6 ounces (¾ cup)

Carrots, 1 bag of baby and 1 small bag of regular size

Chives, 1 bunch

Cilantro, 1 bunch

Cucumber, 2

Dill, 1 bunch

Eggplant, 1 small

Garlic, 12 cloves (3 heads)

Ginger, fresh, 1 medium piece

Green beans, 1 pound

Greens of choice for wilting and salads (kale, spinach, Swiss chard), 2 bunches

Kiwis, 2

Limes, 2

Oranges, 4

Pineapple, 1 small

Raspberries, 1 pint

Red grapes, 1 bunch

Red-skinned potato, 2 medium

Romaine lettuce, 1 head

Scallions, 1 bunch

Spinach, baby leaves, 1 box

Strawberries, 2 pints

Sweet potato, 1 small

Tomatoes, 3 medium

Tomatoes, grape or cherry, 1 pint (use interchangeably)

Tomatoes, diced, 1 can (14.5 ounces; look for brands with no onions or garlic)

Tomatoes, plum, about 1 pound

Zucchini, 2 small

NUTS/SEEDS

Almond flour

Almonds, whole and sliced **

Chia seeds**

Flaxseed, ground**

Peanut butter, all natural (such as Smucker's, Teddie, or 365 Whole Foods)**

Pumpkin seeds**

Sesame seeds**

Sunflower seeds

Walnuts**

SPICES/PANTRY ITEMS

Baking powder

Baking soda

Black pepper, ground**

Brown rice, long-grain, 1 bag

Brown rice couscous, 1 box (look for this in gluten-free section of the grocery store)

Brown rice flour (such as Bob's Red Mill), 1 bag

Cardamom

Chili powder (look for brands with no onion or garlic, such as Spice Appeal)**

Cinnamon**

Coconut milk, light, 1 can or box

Coriander

Corn tortillas, 2 (or more, if prefer to sub for corn tostada shells)

Corn tostada shells, 2

Crackers, brown rice (such as Edward and Sons)

Cumin**

Dark chocolate, 2 ounces

Dijon mustard**

Garlic-infused oil**

Ginger, ground

Gluten-free pasta, 4 ounces

Green olives, 1 jar**

Italian seasoning

Mandarin oranges, 1 small can, in 100% fruit juice

Maple syrup, 100% pure**

Oat bran (such as Bob's Red Mill or Quaker)**

Olive oil**

Paprika**

Peanut oil**

Quinoa, 1 cup**

Red wine vinegar**

Rice vinegar**

Sea salt**

Semisweet chocolate chips, 1 small bag

Sesame oil**

Soy sauce, reduced sodium **

Turmeric**

Vanilla extract or paste**

Notes

Chapter 1

1. Centers for Disease Control and Prevention, National Center for Health Statistics, *Health, United States, 2012: With Special Feature on Emergency Care.* Hyattsville, Maryland (2013), www.cdc.gov/nchs/data/hus/hus12.pdf.

2. M. Tjepkema, "Adult Obesity in Canada: Measured Height and Weight," *Canadian Community Health Survey,* Cat. No. 82-620-MWE, www.statcan.gc.ca/pub/82-620-m/2005001/pdf/4224906-eng.pdf.

3. World Health Organization, "Obesity and Overweight," Fact Sheet N311, March 2013, www.who.int/mediacentre/factsheets/fs311/en/.

4. C. D. Fryar and R. B. Ervin, "Caloric Intake from Fast Food among Adults: United States, 2007–2010," *National Center for Health Statistics Data Brief,* no. 114 (February 2013): 1–7.

5. US Department of Health and Human Services, "Lesson 2: Portion Distortion Presentation," part of the National Heart, Lung, and Blood Institute Obesity education initiative, February 2013.

6. I. H. Steenhuis and W. M. Vermeer, "Portion Size: Review and Framework for Interventions," *International Journal of Behavioral Nutrition and Physical Activity* 6, no. 58 (August 21, 2009).

7. E. S. George, R. R. Rosenkranz, and G. S. Kolt, "Chronic Disease and Sitting Time in Middle-Aged Australian Males: Findings from the 45 and Up Study," *International Journal of Behavioral Nutrition and Physical Activity* 10, no. 20 (February 8, 2013).

8. F. M. Sanches et al., "Waist Circumference and Visceral Fat in CKD: A Cross-Sectional Study," *American Journal of Kidney Disease* 52, no. 1 (July 2008): 66–73.

9. T. Pischon et al., "General and Abdominal Adiposity and Risk of Death in Europe," *New England Journal of Medicine,* no. 359 (November 2008): 2105–20.

10. E. L. Thomas et al., "Excess Body Fat in Obese and Normal-Weight Subjects," *Nutrition Research Reviews* 25, no. 1 (June 2012): 150–61.

11. R. W. Nesto, "Obesity: A Major Component of the Metabolic Syndrome," *Texas Heart Institute Journal* 32, no. 3 (2005): 387–89.

12. I. J. Neeland et al., "Dysfunctional Adiposity and the Risk of Prediabetes and Type 2 Diabetes in Obese Adults," *Journal of the American Medical Association* 308, no. 11 (2012): 1150–59.

13. M. Bardou, A. N. Barkun, and M. Martel, "Obesity and Colorectal Cancer," *Gut* 62, no. 6 (2013): 933–47.

14. M. La Guardia and M. Giammanco, "Breast Cancer and Obesity," *Panminerva Medica* 43, no. 2 (June 2001): 123–33.

15. S. Hardikar et al., "The Role of Tobacco, Alcohol, and Obesity in Neoplastic Progression to Esophageal Adenocarcinoma: A Prospective Study of Barrett's Esophagus," *PLoS One* 8, no. 1 (2013): e52192.

16. L. Taylor, "IBS Drug Market 'Set to More Than Quadruple by 2020,'" *Online Pharma Times*, January 5, 2012.

17. D. Y. Graham, J. L. Smith, and D. J. Patterson, "Why Do Apparently Healthy People Use Antacid Tablets?" *American Journal of Gastroenterology* 78, no. 5 (May 1983): 257–60.

18. U.S. Department of Health and Human Services, "Opportunities and Challenges in Digestive Diseases Research: Recommendations of the National Commission on Digestive Diseases," NIH Publication No. 08-6516 (March 2009).

19. Canadian Digestive Health Foundation, "Digestive Disorders" (2013), www.cdhf.ca/en/disorders.com.

20. Rome Foundation, "Rome III Diagnostic Criteria for Functional Gastrointestinal Disorders," 2006, www.romecriteria.org/assets/pdf/19_RomeIII_apA_885-898.pdf.

21. K. C. Cain et al., "Gender Differences in Gastrointestinal, Psychological, and Somatic Symptoms in Irritable Bowel Syndrome," *Digestive Diseases and Sciences* 54, no. 7 (July 2009): 1542–49.

22. "What Is Morning Sickness? What Causes Morning Sickness?" *Medical News Today*, February 18, 2010. www.medicalnewstoday.com/articles/179633.php

23. National Institutes of Health, "NIH Human Microbiome Project Defines Normal Bacterial Makeup of the Body," news release, June 13, 2012, www.nih.gov/news/health/jun2012/nhgri-13.htm.

24. Ibid.

25. K. E. Scholz-Ahrens et al., "Prebiotics, Probiotics, and Synbiotics Affect Mineral Absorption, Bone Mineral Content, and Bone Structure," supplement, *The Journal of Nutrition* 137, no. 3 (March 2007): S838–S46.

26. A. M. Abdel-Salam et al., "High Fiber Probiotic Fermented Mare's Milk Reduces the Toxic Effects of Mercury in Rats," *North American Journal of Medical Sciences* 2, no. 12 (December 2010): 569–75.

27. L. J. Brandt et al., "An Evidence-Based Position Statement on the Management of Irritable Bowel Syndrome," supplement, *American Journal of Gastroenterology* 104, no. S1 (January 2009): S1–S35.

28. F. Guarner and J. R. Malagelada, "Gut Flora in Health and Disease," *Lancet* 361, no. 9356 (February 2003): 512–19.

29. A. Dukowicz, B. Lacy, and G. Levine, "Small Intestinal Bacterial Overgrowth: A Comprehensive Review," *Gastroenterology and Hepatology* 3, no. 2 (February 2007): 112–22.

30. F. Tsai and W. J. Coyle, "The Microbiome and Obesity: Is Obesity Linked to Our Gut Flora?" *Current Gastroenterology Reports* 11, no. 4 (August 11, 2009): 307–13.

31. R. Mathur et al., "Methane and Hydrogen Positivity on Breath Test Is Associated with Greater Body Mass Index and Body Fat," *The Journal of Clinical Endocrinology & Metabolism* 98, no. 4 (April 2013): E698–702.

32. G. Kim et al., "*Methanobrevibacter Smithii* Is the Predominant Methanogen in Patients with Constipation-Predominant IBS and Methane on Breath," *Digestive Diseases and Sciences* 57, no. 12 (December 2012): 3213–18.

33. M. L. Zupancic et al., "Analysis of the Gut Microbiota in the Old Order Amish and Its Relation to the Metabolic Syndrome," *PLoS One* 7, no. 8 (2012): e43052.

34. J. L. Pluznick et al., "Olfactory Receptor Responding to Gut Microbiota-Derived Signals Plays a Role in Renin Secretion and Blood Pressure Regulation," *Proceedings of the National Academy of Sciences of the United States of America* 110, no. 11 (March 12, 2013): 4410–15.

35. Z. Wang et al., "Gut Flora Metabolism of Phosphatidylcholine Promotes Cardiovascular Disease," *Nature* 472, no. 7341 (April 7, 2011): 57–63.

36. R. A. Koeth et al., "Intestinal Microbiota Metabolism of L-carnitine, a Nutrient in Red Meat, Promotes Atherosclerosis," *Nature Medicine* 19 (2013): 576–85.

37. K. Tillisch et al., "Consumption of Fermented Milk Product with Probiotic Modulates Brain Activity," *Gastroenterology* 144, no. 7 (June 2013): 1394–1401.

38. J. G. Markle et al., "Sex Differences in the Gut Microbiome Drive Hormone-Dependent Regulation of Autoimmunity," *Science* 339, no. 6123 (March 2013): 1084–88.

39. National Institutes of Health, "NIH Human Microbiome Project Defines Normal Bacterial Makeup of the Body," news release, June 13, 2012, www.nih.gov/news/health/jun2012/nhgri-13.htm.

40. G. Vighi et al., "Allergy and the Gastrointestinal System," supplement, *Clinical and Experimental Immunology* 153, no. S1 (September 2008): S3–S6.

41. R. V. Considine et al., "Serum Immunoreactive-Leptin Concentrations in Normal-Weight and Obese Humans," *New England Journal of Medicine* 334, no. 5 (February 1, 1996): 292–95.

42. S. Rakoff-Nahoum, "Why Cancer and Inflammation?" *Yale Journal of Biology and Medicine* 79, nos. 3–4 (December 2006): 123–30.

Chapter 2

1. K. Murakami et al., "Hardness (Difficulty of Chewing) of the Habitual Diet in Relation to Body Mass Index and Waist Circumference in Free-Living Japanese Women Aged 18-22 Y[ears]," *American Journal of Clinical Nutrition* 86, no. 1 (July 2007): 206–13.

2. Y. Zhu and J. Hollis, "Increasing the number of masticatory cycles reduces food intake in healthy young adults," Experimental Biology 2012 Conference, San Diego (April 2012), http://www.aspet.org/uploadedFiles/Meeting/Annual_Meeting/Full%20Program%20for%20Website.pdf

3. A. M. O'Hara and F. Shanahan, "The Gut Flora as a Forgotten Organ," EMBO Reports 7, no. 7 (July 2006): 688–93.

4. R. Mishori, A. Otubu, and A. A. Jones, "The Dangers of Colon Cleansing," *The Journal of Family Practice* 60, no. 8 (August 2011): 454–57.

5. Institute of Medicine, Food and Nutrition Board, *Dietary Reference Intakes for Energy, Carbohydrate, Fiber, Fat, Fatty Acids, Cholesterol, Protein, and Amino Acids* (Washington, D.C.: National Academies Press, 2005).

6. B. L. Pool-Zobel and J. Sauer, "Overview of Experimental Data on Reduction of Colorectal Cancer Risk by Inulin-Type Fructans," supplement, *Journal of Nutrition* 137, no. S11 (November 2007): S580–S84.

7. P. D. Cani et al., "Gut Microbiota Fermentation of Prebiotics Increases Satietogenic and Incretin Gut Peptide Production with Consequences for Appetite Sensation and Glucose Response After a Meal," *American Journal of Clinical Nutrition* 90, no. 5 (November 2009): 1236–43.

8. P. D. Cani et al., "Oligofructose Promotes Satiety in Healthy Human: A Pilot Study," *European Journal of Clinical Nutrition* 60, no. 5 (May 2006): 567–72.

9. J. S. Petrofsky et al., "Muscle Activity During Yoga Breathing Exercise Compared to Abdominal Crunches," *Journal of Applied Research* 5, no. 3 (2005): 501–7.

10. U. C. Ghoshal et al., "Slow Transit Constipation Associated with Excess Methane Production and Its Improvement Following Rifaximin Therapy: A Case Report," *Journal of Neurogastroenterology and Motility* 17, no. 2 (April 2011): 185–88.

11. M. T. Bailey et al., "Exposure to a Social Stressor Alters the Structure of the Intestinal Microbiota: Implications for Stressor-Induced Immunomodulation," *Brain, Behavior, and Immunity* 25, no. 3 (March 2011): 397–407.

12. O. Koren et al., "Host Remodeling of the Gut Microbiome and Metabolic Changes During Pregnancy," *Cell* 150, no. 3 (August 3, 2012): 470–80.

13. R. E. Ley et al., "Microbial Ecology: Human Gut Microbes Associated with Obesity," *Nature* 444 (December 21, 2006): 1022–23.

14. G. D. Wu et al., "Linking Long-Term Dietary Patterns with Gut Microbial Enterotypes," *Science* 334, no. 6052 (October 7, 2011): 105–8.

15. K. Kim et al., "High Fat Diet-Induced Gut Microbiota Exacerbates Inflammation and Obesity in Mice via the TLR4 Signaling Pathway," *PLoS One* 7, no. 10 (2012): e47713.

16. S. Devkota et al., "Dietary-Fat-Induced Taurocholic Acid Promotes Pathobiont Expansion and Colitis in Il10-/- Mice," *Nature* 487 (July 5, 2012): 104–8.

17. S. Cohen et al., "Chronic Stress, Glucocorticoid Receptor Resistance, Inflammation, and Disease Risk," *PNAS* 109, no. 16 (April 17, 2012): 5995–99.

18. J. P. Chaput and A. Tremblay, "Does Short Sleep Duration Favor Abdominal Adiposity in Children?" *International Journal of Pediatric Obesity* 2, no. 3 (2007): 188–91.

19. M. A. Grandner et al., "Dietary Nutrients Associated with Short and Long Sleep Duration: Data from a Nationally Representative Sample," *Appetite* 64 (May 2013): 71–80.

20. T. Deng et al., "Class II Major Histocompatibility Complex Plays an Essential Role in Obesity-Induced Adipose Inflammation," *Cell Metabolism* 17, no. 3 (March 5, 2013): 411–22.

21. P. Cani et al., "Changes in Gut Microbiota Control Metabolic Endotoxemia-Induced Inflammation in High-Fat Diet–Induced Obesity and Diabetes in Mice," *Diabetes* 57, no. 6 (June 2008): 1470–81.

22. E. A. Schwartz et al., "Nutrient Modification of the Innate Immune Response: A Novel Mechanism by Which Saturated Fatty Acids Greatly Amplify Monocyte Inflammation," *Arteriosclerosis, Thrombosis, and Vascular Biology* 30, no. 4 (April 2010): 802–8.

23. D. Mozaffarian et al., "Dietary Intake of Trans Fatty Acids and Systemic Inflammation in Women," *American Journal of Clinical Nutrition* 79, no. 4 (April 2004): 606–12.

24. A. P. Simopoulos, "The Importance of the Ratio of Omega-6/Omega-3 Essential Fatty Acids," *Biomedicine & Pharmacotherapy* 56, no. 8 (October 2002): 365–79.

25. J. Bures et al., "Small Intestinal Bacterial Overgrowth Syndrome," *World Journal of Gastroenterology* 16, no. 24 (June 28, 2010): 2978–90.

26. E. Walderhaug et al., "Interactive Effects of Sex and 5-HTTLPR on Mood and Impulsivity During Tryptophan Depletion in Healthy People," *Biological Psychiatry* 62, no. 6 (September 15, 2007): 593–99.

27. I. Spreadbury, "Comparison with Ancestral Diets Suggests Dense Acellular Carbohydrates Promote an Inflammatory Microbiota, and May Be the Primary Dietary Cause of Leptin Resistance and Obesity," *Diabetes, Metabolic Syndrome and Obesity: Targets and Therapy* 5 (2012): 175–89.

28. M. Osterdahl et al., "Effects of a Short-Term Intervention with a Paleolithic Diet in Healthy Volunteers," *European Journal of Clinical Nutrition* 62, no. 5 (May 2008): 682–85.

29. L. A. Frassetto et al., "Metabolic and Physiologic Improvements from Consuming a Paleolithic, Hunter-Gatherer Type Diet," *European Journal of Clinical Nutrition* 63, no. 8 (August 2009): 947–55.

30. T. Jönsson et al., "Beneficial Effects of a Paleolithic Diet on Cardiovascular Risk Factors in Type 2 Diabetes: A Randomized Cross-Over Pilot Study," *Cardiovascular Diabetology* 8 (July 16, 2009): 35.

31. S. Lindeberg et al., "A Paleolithic Diet Improves Glucose Tolerance More Than a Mediterranean-Like Diet in Individuals with Ischaemic Heart Disease," *Diabetologia* 50, no. 9 (September 2007): 1795–1807.

32. T. Jönsson et al., "A Paleolithic Diet Is More Satiating per Calorie Than a Mediterranean-Like Diet in Individuals with Ischemic Heart Disease," *Nutrition & Metabolism* 7 (November 2010): 85.

33. R. J. Wurtman et al., "Effects of Normal Meals Rich in Carbohydrates or Proteins on Plasma Tryptophan and Tyrosine Ratios," *American Journal of Clinical Nutrition* 77, no. 1 (January 2003): 128–32.

34. A. K. Campbell et al., "Bacterial Metabolic 'Toxins': A New Mechanism for Lactose and Food Intolerance, and Irritable Bowel Syndrome," *Toxicology* 278, no. 3 (December 2010): 268–76.

35. A. Sapone, et al., "Divergence of Gut Permeability and Mucosal Immune Gene Expression in Two Gluten-Associated Conditions: Celiac Disease and Gluten Sensitivity," *BMC Medicine* 9, no. 23 (2011).

36. J. S. Barrett and P. R. Gibson, "Fermentable Oligosaccharides, Disaccharides, Monosaccharides and Polyols (FODMAPs) and Nonallergic Food Intolerance: FODMAPs or Food Chemicals?" *Therapeutic Advances in Gastroenterology* 5, no. 4 (July 2012): 261–68.

37. R. Gearry et al., "Reduction of Dietary Poorly Absorbed Short-Chain Carbohydrates (FODMAPs) Improves Abdominal Symptoms in Patients with Inflammatory Bowel Disease—A Pilot Study," *Journal of Crohn's and Colitis* 3, no. 1 (February 2009): 8–14.

Chapter 3

1. M. Levitt et al., "Belching, Bloating and Flatulence," American College of Gastroenterology (June 2004), http://s3.gi.org/patients/gihealth/pdf/belching.pdf.

2. B. Lacy et al., "Pathophysiology, Evaluation, and Treatment of Bloating," *Gastroenterology & Hepatology* 7, no. 11 (November 2011): 729–39.

3. R. J. Basseri et al., "Antibiotics for the Treatment of Irritable Bowel Syndrome," *Gastroenterology & Hepatology* 7, no. 7 (July 2011): 455–93.

4. National Institutes of Health, "Gas in the Digestive Track," National Digestive Diseases Information Clearinghouse Publication No. 13-883, November 2012.

5. F. Suarez, J. Springfield, and M. Levitt, "Identification of Gases Responsible for the Odour of Human Flatus and Evaluation of a Device Purported to Reduce This Odour," *Gut* 43, no. 1 (July 1998): 100–104.

6. National Institutes of Health, "Heartburn, Gastroesophageal Reflux (GER), and Gastroesophageal Reflux Disease (GERD)," National Digestive Diseases Information Clearinghouse Publication No. 07-0882 (May 2007).

7. Canadian Digestive Health Foundation, "Your Digestive Health," May 2010, www.cdhf.ca/en/disorders/details/id/11.

8. J. Everhart, "The Burden of Digestive Diseases in the United States," National Digestive Diseases Information Clearinghouse Publication No. 09-6443, 2008.

9. F. K. Friedenberg et al., "Trends in Gastroesophageal Reflux Disease as Measured by the National Ambulatory Medical Care Survey," *Digestive Diseases and Sciences* 55, no. 7 (July 2010): 1911–17.

10. G. Karamanolis et al., "A Glass of Water Immediately Increases Gastric pH in Healthy Subjects," *Digestive Diseases and Sciences* 53, no. 12 (December 2008): 3128–32.

11. J. Dent et al., "Epidemiology of Gastro-Oesophageal Disease: A Systematic Review," *Gut* 54, no. 5 (May 2005): 710–17.

12. D. Compare et al., "Effects of Long-Term PPI Treatment on Producing Bowel Symptoms and SIBO," *European Journal of Clinical Investigations* 41, no. 4 (April 2011): 380–86.

13. A. J. Eherer et al., "Positive Effect of Abdominal Breathing Exercise on Gastroesophageal Reflux Disease: A Randomized, Controlled Study," *American Journal of Gastroenterology* 107, no. 3 (March 2012): 372–78.

14. N. Talley, "Chronic Constipation May Increase Risk of Colorectal Cancer, Benign Neoplasms," presented at the American College of Gastroenterology 77th annual scientific meeting, October 2012.

15. P. D. Higgins and J. F. Johanson, "Epidemiology of Constipation in North America: A Systematic Review," *American Journal of Gastroenterology* 99, no. 4 (April 2004): 750–59.

16. J. A. Marlett, T. M. Kajs, and M. H. Fischer, "An Unfermented Gel Component of Psyllium Seed Husk Promotes Laxation as a Lubricant in Humans," *American Journal of Clinical Nutrition* 72, no. 3 (September 2000): 784–89.

17. H. L. Chen et al., "Mechanisms by Which Wheat Bran and Oat Bran Increase Stool Weight in Humans," *American Journal of Clinical Nutrition* 68, no. 3 (September 1998): 711–19.

18. J. Slavin and J. Feirtag, "Chicory Inulin Does Not Increase Stool Weight or Speed Up Intestinal Transit Time in Healthy Male Subjects," *Food & Function* 2, no. 1 (January 2011): 72–7.

19. U.S. Department of Agriculture and U.S. Department of Health and Human Services, *Dietary Guidelines for Americans, 2010*, 7th edition (Washington, DC: U.S. Government Printing Office, 2010).

20. H. L. DuPont, "Guidelines on Acute Infectious Diarrhea in Adults," *The American Journal of Gastroenterology* 92, no. 11 (November 1997): 1962–75.

21. L. R. Schiller, "Chronic Diarrhea," *Gastroenterology* 127, no. 1 (July 2004): 287–93.

22. Basseri et al., "Antibiotics for the Treatment," 729–39.

23. R. Mattar, D. F. de Campos Mazo, and F. J. Carrilho, "Lactose Intolerance: Diagnosis, Genetic, and Clinical Factors," *Clinical and Experimental Gastroenterology* 5 (2012): 113–21.

24. University of Maryland Medical Center, "University of Maryland School of Medicine Researchers Identify Key Pathogenic Differences between Celiac Disease and Gluten Sensitivity," news release, March 10, 2011, http://www.umm.edu/news/releases/gluten-sensitivity-celiac-disease.htm#ixzz2U1XCd3cP

25. A. Rubio-Tapia et al., "The Prevalence of Celiac Disease in the United States," *American Journal of Gastroenterology* 107, no. 10 (October 2012): 1538–44.

26. A. Rubio-Tapia et al., "Increased Prevalence and Mortality in Undiagnosed Celiac Disease," *Gastroenterology* 137, no. 1 (July 2009): 88–93.

27. S. G. Park et al., "Effects of Rehydration Fluid Temperature and Composition on Body Weight Retention upon Voluntary Drinking Following Exercise-Induced Dehydration," *Nutrition Research and Practice* 6, no. 2 (April 2012): 126–31.

28. Q. Zhou and G. N. Verne, "New Insights into Visceral Hypersensitivity—Clinical Implications in IBS," *Nature Reviews: Gastroenterology & Hepatology* 8, no. 6 (June 2011): 349–55.

29. Canadian Digestive Health Foundation, "Your Digestive Health."

30. S. Thevarajah et al., "Hormonal Influences on the Gastrointestinal Tract and Irritable Bowel Syndrome," *Practical Gastroenterology* (May 2005): 62–74.

31. E. A. Mayer et al., "Stress and the Gastrointestinal Tract," *American Journal of Physiology-Gastrointestinal and Liver Physiology* 280, no. 4 (April 2001): G519–24.

32. W. D. Heizer, S. Southern, and S. McGovern, "The Role of Diet in Symptoms of Irritable Bowel Syndrome in Adults: A Narrative Review," *Journal of the American Dietetic Association* 109, no. 7 (July 2009): 1204–14.

33. Y. Sun et al., "Stress-Induced Corticotropin-Releasing Hormone-Mediated NLRP6 Inflammasome Inhibition and Transmissible Enteritis in Mice," *Gastroenterology* 144, no. 7 (June 2013): 1478–87.

34. J. Rouse, "Nutritional Management of Irritable Bowel Syndrome: A Summary," *Advanced Nutrition Publications* (2002).

Chapter 4

1. I. Aeberli, "Low to Moderate Sugar-Sweetened Beverage Consumption Impairs Glucose and Lipid Metabolism and Promotes Inflammation in Healthy Young Men: A Randomized Controlled Trial," *American Journal of Clinical Nutrition* 94, no. 2 (August 2011): 479–85.

2. L. C. Hudgins, "Effect of High-Carbohydrate Feeding on Triglyceride and Saturated Fatty Acid Synthesis," *Proceedings of the Society for Experimental Biology and Medicine* 225, no. 3 (December 2000): 178–83.

3. U. N. Prakash and K. Srinivasan, "Fat Digestion and Absorption in Spice-Pretreated Rats," *Journal of the Science of Food and Agriculture,* September 14, 2011.

4. National Cancer Institute, "Risk Factor Monitoring and Methods: Table 1. Top Food Sources of Saturated Fat Among US Population, 2005–2006," from the National Health and Nutrition Examination Survey, http://riskfactor.cancer.gov/diet/foodsources/sat_fat/sf.html.

5. D. M. Swallow, "Genetics of Lactase Persistence and Lactose Intolerance," *Annual Review of Genetics* 37 (December 2003): 197–219.

6. T. Bersaglieri et al., "Genetic Signatures of Strong Recent Positive Selection at the Lactase Gene," *American Journal of Human Genetics* 74, no. 6 (June 2004): 1111–20.

7. T. He et al., "Effects of Yogurt and Bifidobacteria Supplementation on the Colonic Microbiota in Lactose-Intolerant Subjects," *Journal of Applied Microbiology* 104, no. 2 (February 2008): 595–604.

8. Y. K. Choi et al., "Fructose Intolerance in IBS and Utility of Fructose-Restricted Diet," *Journal of Clinical Gastroenterology* 42, no. 3 (March 2008): 233–38.

9. M. E. Bocarsly et al., "High-Fructose Corn Syrup Causes Characteristics of Obesity in Rats: Increased Body Weight, Body Fat and Triglyceride Levels," *Pharmacology, Biochemistry, and Behavior* 97, no. 1 (November 2010): 101–6.

10. K. L. Stanhope et al., "Consuming Fructose-Sweetened, not Glucose-Sweetened, Beverages Increases Visceral Adiposity and Lipids and Decreases Insulin Sensitivity in Overweight/Obese Humans," *Journal of Clinical Investigation* 119, no. 5 (May 2009): 1322–34.

11. M. Song et al., "High Fructose Feeding Induces Copper Deficiency in Sprague-Dawley Rats: A Novel Mechanism for Obesity Related Fatty Liver," *Journal of Hepatology* 56, no. 2 (February 2012): 433–40.

12. United States Department of Agriculture, "Sugar and Sweeteners Outlook, NAFTA and World Sugar June 2013," Economic Research Service, June 18, 2013, http://www.ers.usda.gov/media/1131601/sssm298.pdf

13. Sue Shepherd and Peter Gibson, *The Complete Low-FODMAP Diet* (The Experiment, 2013).

14. H. A. Grabitske and J. L. Slavin, "Gastrointestinal Effects of Low-Digestible Carbohydrates," *Critical Reviews in Food Science and Nutrition* 49, no. 4 (April 2009): 327–60.

15. M. B. Abou-Donia et al., "Splenda Alters Gut Microflora and Increases Intestinal P-Glycoprotein and Cytochrome P-450 in Male Rats," *Journal of Toxicology and Environmental Health, Part A* 71, no. 21 (2008): 1415–29.

16. Fde. M. Feijo et al., "Saccharin and Aspartame, Compared with Sucrose, Induce Greater Weight Gain in Adult Wistar Rats, at Similar Total Caloric Intakes," *Appetite* 60, no. 1 (January 2013): 203–07.

Chapter 5

1. F. H. Nielsen, "Magnesium, Inflammation, and Obesity in Chronic Disease," *Nutrition Reviews* 68, no. 6 (June 2010): 333–40.

2. K. M. Elias et al., "Retinoic Acid Inhibits Th17 Polarization and Enhances FoxP3 Expression Through a Stat-3/Stat-5 Independent Signaling Pathway," *Blood* 111, no. 3 (February 2008): 1013–20.

3. C. S. Johnston et al., "Plasma Vitamin C Is Inversely Related to Body Mass Index and Waist Circumference but Not to Plasma Adiponectin in Nonsmoking Adults," *Journal of Nutrition* 137, no. 7 (July 2007): 1757–62.

4. R. P. Heaney and C. M. Weaver, "Calcium Absorption from Kale," *American Journal of Clinical Nutrition* 51, no. 4 (April 1990): 656–57.

5. R. YanardaÐ and H. Çolak, "Effect of Chard (*Beta vulgaris* L. var. cicla) on Blood Glucose Levels in Normal and Alloxan-Induced Diabetic Rabbits," *Pharmacy and Pharmacology Communications* 4, no. 6 (June 1998): 309–11.

6. L. Cloetens et al., "Role of Dietary Beta-Glucans in the Prevention of the Metabolic Syndrome," *Nutrition Reviews* 70, no. 8 (August 2012): 444–58.

7. K. C. Maki et al., "Whole-Grain Ready-to-Eat Oat Cereal, as Part of a Dietary Program for Weight Loss, Reduces Low-Density Lipoprotein Cholesterol in Adults with Overweight and Obesity More Than a Dietary Program Including Low-Fiber Control Foods," *Journal of the American Dietetic Association* 110, no. 2 (February 2010): 205–14.

8. C. J. Traoret et al., "Peanut Digestion and Energy Balance," *International Journal of Obesity* 32, no. 2 (February 2008): 322–28.

9. R. Wall et al., "Fatty Acids from Fish: The Anti-Inflammatory Potential of Long-Chain Omega-3 Fatty Acids," *Nutrition Reviews* 68, no. 5 (May 2010): 280–89.

10. F. Fernández-Bañares et al., "Changes in Mucosal Fatty Acid Profile in Inflammatory Bowel Disease and in Experimental Colitis: A Common Response to Bowel Inflammation," *Clinical Nutrition* 16, no. 4 (August 1997): 177–83.

11. J. A. Paniagua et al., "Monounsaturated Fat-Rich Diet Prevents Central Body Fat Distribution and Decreases Postprandial Adiponectin Expression Induced by a Carbohydrate-Rich Diet in Insulin-Resistant Subjects," *Diabetes Care* 30, no. 7 (2007): 1717–23.

12. P. Schieberle et al., "Identifying Substances That Regulate Satiety in Oils and Fats and Improving Low-Fat Foodstuffs by Adding Lipid Compounds with a High Satiety Effect; Key Findings of the DFG/AiF cluster project 'Perception of Fat Content and Regulating Satiety: An Approach to Developing Low-Fat Foodstuffs,'" 2009–2012, www.tum.de/en/about-tum/news/press-releases/short/article/30517/.

13. E. M. Evans et al., "Effects of Protein Intake and Gender on Body Composition Changes: A Randomized Clinical Weight Loss Trial," *Nutrition & Metabolism* 9, no. 1 (June 2012): 55.

14. C. S. Johnston, S. L. Tjonn, and P. D. Swan, "High-Protein, Low-Fat Diets Are Effective for Weight Loss and Favorably Alter Biomarkers in Healthy Adults," *Journal of Nutrition* 134, no. 3 (March 2004): 586–91.

15. M. B. Zemel et al., "Dairy Augmentation of Total and Central Fat Loss in Obese Subjects," *International Journal of Obesity* 29, no. 4 (April 2005): 391–97.

16. D. I. Batovska et al., "Antibacterial Study of the Medium Chain Fatty Acids and Their 1-Monoglycerides: Individual Effects and Synergistic Relationships," *Polish Journal of Microbiology* 58, no. 1 (2009): 43–7.

17. S. Lieberman, M. G. Enig, and H. G. Preuss, "A Review of Monolaurin and Lauric Acid: Natural Virucidal and Bactericidal Agents," *Alternative and Complementary Therapies* 12, no. 6 (December 2006): 310–14.

18. K. L. Wu et al., "Effects of Ginger on Gastric Emptying and Motility in Healthy Humans," *European Journal of Gastroenterology and Hepatology* 20, no. 5 (May 2008): 436–40.

19. F. Ke, et al., "Herbal Medicine in the Treatment of Ulcerative Colitis," *Saudi Journal of Gastroenterology* 18, no. 1 (January–February 2012): 3–10.

20. S. Kumar et al., "Curcumin for Maintenance of Remission in Ulcerative Colitis," *Cochrane Database of Systematic Reviews* 10 (October 17, 2012).

Chapter 6

1. B. Sears and C. Ricordi, "Anti-Inflammatory Nutrition as a Pharmacological Approach to Treat Obesity," *Journal of Obesity* 2011 (2011): article ID 431985. Published online 2010 September 30. doi: 10.1155/2011/431985

Chapter 8

1. T. S. Church et al., "Changes in Weight, Waist Circumference and Compensatory Responses with Different Doses of Exercise Among Sedentary, Overweight Postmenopausal Women," *PLoS One* 4, no. 2 (2009): e4515.

2. J. C. Marshall, "The Gut as a Potential Trigger of Exercise-Induced Inflammatory Responses," *Canadian Journal of Physiology and Pharmacology* 76, no. 5 (May 1998): 479–84.

3. E. P. de Oliveira and R. C. Burini, "The Impact of Physical Exercise on the Gastrointestinal Tract," *Current Opinion in Clinical Nutrition and Metabolic Care* 12, no. 5 (September 2009): 533–38.

4. F. M. Moses, "The Effect of Exercise on the Gastrointestinal Tract," *Sports Medicine* 9, no. 3 (March 1990): 159–72.

5. J. C. Murphy et al., "Preferential Reductions in Intermuscular and Visceral Adipose Tissue with Exercise-Induced Weight Loss Compared with Calorie Restriction," *Journal of Applied Physiology* 112, no. 1 (January 2012): 79–85.

6. M. Ayabe et al., "Accumulation of Short Bouts of Non-Exercise Daily Physical Activity Is Associated with Lower Visceral Fat in Japanese Female Adults," *International Journal of Sports Medicine* 34, no. 1 (January 2013): 62–7.

7. V. A. Catenacci et al., "Physical Activity Patterns in the National Weight Control Registry," *Obesity* 16, no. 1 (January 2008): 153–61.

8. E. Johannesson et al., "Physical Activity Improves Symptoms in Irritable Bowel Syndrome: A Randomized Controlled Trial," *American Journal of Gastroenterology* 106, no. 5 (May 2011): 915–22.

9. K. Ogawa et al., "Resistance Exercise Training-Induced Muscle Hypertrophy Was Associated with Reduction of Inflammatory Markers in Elderly Women," *Mediators of Inflammation* (2010), doi:10.1155/2010/171023.

10. L. A. Daray et al., "Endurance and Resistance Training Lowers C-Reactive Protein in Young, Healthy Females," *Applied Physiology, Nutrition, and Metabolism* 36, no. 5 (October 2011): 660–70.

11. A. Dietrich and W. F. McDaniel, "Endocannabinoids and Exercise," *British Journal of Sports Medicine* 38, no. 5 (October 2004): 536–41.

12. S. H. Boutcher, "High-Intensity Intermittent Exercise and Fat Loss," *Journal of Obesity* (2011), doi: 10.1155/2011/868305.

13. D. R. Broom et al., "Exercise-Induced Suppression of Acylated Ghrelin in Humans," *Journal of Applied Physiology* 102, no. 6 (June 2007): 2165–71.

14. P. Boudou et al., "Absence of Exercise-Induced Variations in Adiponectin Levels Despite Decreased Abdominal Adiposity and Improved Insulin Sensitivity in Type 2 Diabetic Men," *European Journal of Endocrinology* 149, no. 5 (November 2003): 421–24.

15. A. Mourier et al., "Mobilization of Visceral Adipose Tissue Related to the Improvement in Insulin Sensitivity in Response to Physical Training in NIDD," *Diabetes Care* 20, no. 3 (March 1997): 385–91.

16. J. Mager et al., "The Influence of Classical Yoga Practices on Plasma Cortisol Levels," presented at the 85th meeting of the Endocrine Society, 2003.

17. R. K. Yadav et al., "Efficacy of a Short-Term Yoga-Based Lifestyle Intervention in Reducing Stress and Inflammation: Preliminary Results," *Journal of Alternative and Complementary Medicine* 18, no. 7 (July 2012): 662–67.

18. I Taneja et al., "Yogic Versus Conventional Treatment in Diarrhea-Predominant Irritable Bowel Syndrome: A Randomized Control Study," *Applied Psychophysiology and Biofeedback* 29, no. 1 (March 2004): 19–33.

19. L. Kuttner et al., "A Randomized Trial of Yoga for Adolescents with Irritable Bowel Syndrome," *Pain Research & Management* 11, no. 4 (Winter 2006): 217–24.

20. J. Hermann, T. Kościński, and M. Drews, "Practical Approach to Constipation in Adults," *Ginekologia Polska* 83, no. 11 (November 2012): 849–53.

Chapter 9

1. T. N. Akbaraly et al., "Dietary Pattern and Depressive Symptoms in Middle Age," *British Journal of Psychiatry* 195, no. 5 (November 2009): 408–13.

Index

Curried Chicken Soup, 164

Green Beans Amandine, 214

Hearty Roasted Vegetable Soup, 168

Grilled Chicken, Sweet Potato, and Kiwi Salad, 191

Grilled Turkey Cutlets with Grape Salsa, 172

gut (GI tract), 7, 233

gut bacteria

body weight link, 14–16, 31

causes of imbalance in, 30–33, 37

disease link, 16–17

inflammation and, 16, 35

term, 10

gut flora. *See* gut bacteria

gut microbiota. *See* gut bacteria

H

happiness, 262–263

hazelnuts, 101–102

HCL, 26–27

heart attack, 57

heartburn, 55–60

heart disease, 17, 20, 78

Hearty Roasted Vegetable Soup, 168

hemorrhoids, 61, 62

Herb-Roasted Shrimp, 197

hiatal hernia, 56–57

high-fructose corn syrup, 81–83, 84, 257

histamine antagonists, 60

Hoffman, Jamie, 32

Homemade Chicken Broth, 165

honey, 84, 257

honeydew, 99

hormone replacement therapy (HRT), 57

hot sauce, 121

HRT, 57

Human Microbiome Project, 15

hunger, 120, 232, 235

hydration, 62, 64, 68. *See also* water, as remedy

hydrochloric acid (HCL), 26–27

hyperthyroidism, 64

hypnotherapy, 71

hypothyroidism, 62

I

IBD, 19–20, 51

IBS. *See* irritable bowel syndrome

immune system, 17–19, 65

Imodium, 68

individual differences

FODMAPs sensitivity, 44–45

hot sauce sensitivity, 121

lactose intolerance, 80

infections, 31, 34, 64

inflammation

body weight link, 19–20, 34–35

causes of, 33–36, 37, 43–44, 94, 114

defined, 19

disease link, 20

exercise effects on, 234, 237, 238

gut bacteria and, 16, 35

inflammatory bowel disease (IBD), 19–20, 51

insulin, 34

insulin resistance, 37, 82

interval walking, 235–236

intestinal obstructions, 53

inulin, 62, 85

irritable bowel syndrome (IBS)

causes and treatments, 69–71

FODMAPs and, 43

sales of medication for, 7

signs and symptoms, 61, 69

treatments for, 46

isomalt, 90

Italian Swiss Chard, 210

K

kale

as Belly Buddy, 96

Caldo Verde, 166

Kale Caesar Salad, 206

Parmesan-Crumbed Kale, 213

kasha, 181

kefir, 43

kemchi, 43

kiwifruit

as Belly Buddy, 99

Grilled Chicken, Sweet Potato, and Kiwi Salad, 191

Kiwi-Glazed Turkey Meat Loaf, 173

L

lactase supplements, 54, 257

lactose, 79–81, 257

lactose intolerance

lactose tolerance limits, 45, 51, 80

misdiagnosis, 28

rates of, 65

large intestine, 26

lauric acid, 107

laxatives, 53, 63, 65

leeks, 85

legumes, 85

omega-6 fats
  as Belly Bully, 78, 79
  inflammation link, 35–36,
    103–104
onions
  as Belly Bully, 85
  cooking without, 84–85,
    121–122
  gas from, 53
  testing, 258
oranges
  as Belly Buddy, 59, 99
  Creamside Smoothie, 157
  Pork Satay Salad, 186
ovarian cancer, 53

P

packaged foods, 79
Paleo diets, 39
pancreatitis, 64
papaya
  as Belly Buddy, 99
  Pork Satay Salad, 186
Paprika-Spiced Fish Cakes, 180
parasites, 64
Parkinson's disease, 62
Parmesan-Crumbed Kale, 213
parsnips
  as Belly Buddy, 97
  Hearty Roasted Vegetable
    Soup, 168
  Vegetarian Shepherd's Pie,
    199–200
pasta
  Baked Pork Tetrazzini, 188
  as Belly Bully, 77
  Sesame Pasta, 221
  "Caprese" Pasta Salad, 195
peaches, 85, 90, 258
peanuts, peanut butter

as Belly Buddy, 101, 102
Chunky Chocolate Smoothie,
  157
Crunchy Chopped Salad,
  202
Curried Chicken Soup, 164
Kiwi-Glazed Turkey Meat
  Loaf, 173
Peanut Butter–Banana
  Freeze, 226
Crunchy Chicken Couscous,
  192
Pork Satay Salad, 186
Sesame Pasta, 221
pears
  as Belly Bully, 84, 90
  gas from, 53
  test results and, 257, 258
pecans
  as Belly Buddy, 102
  Chipotle Veggie Burgers, 181
  Nutty Red Quinoa, 220
pelvic floor exercises, 241
Pepcid, 60
peptic ulcers, 51, 57
Pepto-Bismol, 59
persimmons, 85
phases of diet, 116–117. *See also*
  Flatten (Phase 1), Soothe
  and Shrink (Phase 2), *and*
  Balance (Phase 3)
pineapple
  as Belly Buddy, 99
  Curry-Rubbed Chicken with
    Fresh Pineapple Chutney,
    174
  Nutty Red Quinoa, 220
pine nuts
  Arugula Pesto Chicken, 176
  as Belly Buddy, 102
pistachios, 85, 101
pizza, 78, 79
plums, 90, 258

polenta, 100
polydextrose, 90
polyols, 89–90, 258
pork
  Baked Pork Tetrazzini, 188
  as Belly Buddy, 106
  Pork Satay Salad, 186
portion size, 3–4
potassium, 98
potatoes
  as Belly Buddy, 97
  Caldo Verde, 166
  carb density of, 37–38
  Hearty Roasted Vegetable
    Soup, 168
  Lemony Salmon, Potato, and
    Dill Bake, 194
  Paprika-Spiced Fish Cakes,
    180
  Ratatouille Frittata, 182
  Twice-Baked Potatoes with
    Pepper Hash, 219
  Vegetarian Shepherd's Pie,
    199–200
poultry, 106
prebiotics, 29
pregnancy, 9, 31, 62
pretzels, 77
Prevacid, 60
Prilosec, 60
probiotics, 15, 31, 71
Procardia, 57
processed meats, 79
pro-inflammatory fats, 77–79
protein, 59, 105–106, 261
proton pump inhibitors, 60
prunes, 90
psyllium seed husk, 62
pumpkin seeds
  as Belly Buddy, 102–103
  Curried Chicken Soup, 164

V

Valium, 57

vegetable oils, 79. *See also* olive
oil

vegetables. *See also specific
vegetables*

Belly Buddies, 96–97

Belly Bullies, 84, 85, 90

Hearty Roasted Vegetable
Soup, 168

in maintenance plan, 260

vegetarian foods

Chipotle Veggie Burgers, 181

substitutions, 105

Vegetarian Shepherd's Pie,
199–200

viruses, 64

visceral fat. *See* belly fat

vitamin B6, 98

vitamin C, 96

W

waist circumference, 5

walking, 235–236

walnuts

as Belly Buddy, 101–102, 105

Grape and Walnut Waldorf
Salad, 204

Multigrain Hot Cereal with
Maple Nuts, 161

Vegetarian She pherd's Pie,
199–200

water, as remedy, 59, 120. *See
also* dehydration

water chestnuts

as Belly Buddy, 97

Crunchy Chopped Salad,
202

watercress, 97

watermelon, 84, 85, 90

water retention, 53–54

weight. *See* body weight;
obesity

weight loss, for heartburn, 60

weight maintenance, 259–262

Weiss, Lauren, 146–147, 266

wheat, 84, 85, 258

wheat bran, 62

Worcestershire Sauce, 153

X

xylitol, 90

Y

yellow squash, 215

yoga, 238, 249–251

yogurt, 68, 81, 153. *See also*
Greek yogurt

Z

Zantac, 60

Zegerid, 60

zucchini

as Belly Buddy, 97

Chipotle Veggie Burgers, 181

Crunchy Chicken Couscous,
192

Ratatouille Frittata, 182

Summer Squash Gratin, 215